If men... ...*!*

Are hot flashes safe? NO!

Is the WHI wrong? YES!

Should women take estrogen lifelong? YES!

Does estrogen replacement prevent Alzheimer's disease and heart disease? YES!

Will my chances decrease of getting breast cancer if I do not take estrogen? NO!

Estrogen Revisited: Lifelong & Fearless

Donna Walters and Blane Crandall, MD

authorHOUSE®

AuthorHouse™
1663 Liberty Drive, Suite 200
Bloomington, IN 47403
www.authorhouse.com
Phone: 1-800-839-8640

First published by AuthorHouse 3/30/2010

ISBN: 978-1-4343-5984-1 (sc)

Library of Congress Control Number: 2007910386

Printed in the United States of America
Bloomington, Indiana

This book is printed on acid-free paper.

Cover photograph of Donna Walters by Alev Sezer-Jacobs.
Additional images of Donna Walters by Rider Photographies.

2nd Edition

Acknowledgements

Donna's

I would like to thank my family and friends for their help, support, and encouragement during the writing of this book. I especially appreciate David, my husband of more than forty-three years, for providing me with very important ideas, constant encouragement and the enthusiasm to keep me on task, and for his patience, critique, artwork and editorial help during the two years that it took to write this book. My children, Dave, Karrie and Chuck, and my daughters-in-law, Dana and Valerie, gave me their full support and interest. I also want to acknowledge my co-workers, Benton Burroughs, Jr., who gave me suggestions, assistance and support along the way, and Sharon Hilliard, who lent an important helping hand and shared both my joy and pain of many revisions. I'd like to give recognition to Marilyn Kentz for her work in making this second edition an enjoyable experience for me. My relatives and close friends in Texas gave me encouragement and reinforced the importance of the book. And lastly, I would like to thank my co-author, Blane Crandall, M.D., for his support and effort with this book in an attempt to right the terrible wrongs concerning women's important health issues.

Blane's

First, I would like to thank Doshie, my wife of almost forty years, for her love and encouragement in all of my pursuits. My son, Blane Mitchell Crandall, M.D., has shared my passion for rectifying this social injustice and he has cared for my patients when I have needed to be away from my medical practice. My son, Roger, has drawn and reconfigured my charts and graphs during many midnight sessions over the past year. I am forever indebted to my parents, Jean and Clarence Crandall, M.D., for giving me the love of learning and the strength to stand firm in my convictions. I could not have made this journey without the support and encouragement of my daughters, Leigh and Kristin. I do appreciate my medical staff, especially Betsy, my assistant for seventeen years, for copying thousands of pages of literature on this topic and keeping patients calm when I ran late during office hours in my attempt to save women one patient at a time since this nonsense started in 2002. Thanks to my friends Duane and Linda Black for editing my notes and taking my photo for this publication. Finally, I must thank Donna Walters for being the impetus to get this project launched and for the confidence that she has placed in me to share the authorship of this book.

Table of Contents

Preface

Donna Walters

At the turn of the twentieth century millions of women all over the world experienced the benefits of hormone replacement therapy (HRT). Many husbands were happy, too. Replacing the depleting estrogen seemed to make their wives feel energetic, sexually playful and in good spirits. Gone were the night sweats, cranky moods, hot flashes and insomnia. The belief during that time: HRT was doing the double-duty of preventing heart disease, osteoporosis and even breast cancer. It was the anti-aging miracle we had all been waiting for. Then, in 2002, came the Women's Health Initiative (WHI) to squash our euphoria.

The WHI declared that women taking hormones could instead be *increasing* their risk for heart disease and breast cancer. Women all over the nation panicked, had a good cry and dropped the program like a hot spud. I was not one of them. Instead, I began a quest: researching further in order to make a more informed decision. As a result, I have vowed that I will never, ever experience menopause.

That initial WHI announcement, though inaccurate and misinterpreted, is still causing confusion and fear today. It is time to reignite estrogen awareness, understand its importance and effects on our health throughout our entire lives — and not just the menopausal years. It's time we make an educated choice about our bodies. Sound familiar? It should. Over forty years ago we finally got the chance to decide when, and if, we would get pregnant. The birth control pill gave women a kind of freedom and power we had never before experienced. And like choosing to replace diminishing estrogen now, it did not come without its risks. The difference in the HRT alternative is that choosing to go through natural menopause comes with just as many, if not more, hazards that could be life altering.

A *great disservice* is being done to women regarding hormone replacement therapy — we are not given *all* of the important medical information concerning our bodies. The fact that we are not provided this information in a timely manner prevents us from making decisions concerning our lifetime health. How unfortunate that many women are not thoroughly informed about the aging process that takes place; what happens during that time period; and most importantly, what can be done to change or slow it down.

The message I want women to get from this book is that menopause has NOT had any improvements EVER! We have the right to a thorough study and a full disclosure regarding the use of hormone replacement therapy versus nature. Inasmuch as nothing has been forthcoming since the sixties regarding estrogen, and there are more than twenty-two negative health consequences for going through this natural, radical change of life, menopause should NOW become a woman's choice. We have the right to choose.

Interestingly, men do not experience aging in the same manner as women; they do not undergo a major chemistry change similar to that of aging females. My father once told me, "Men become distinguished as they age, but unfortunately, women just get old." This "old lady syndrome" can be prevented — and I'm not talking about just appearances. Any woman can get her skin pulled. I am a woman over sixty-two years old who has been taking estrogen for more than thirty years. I am young in appearance, young in spirit, and young in health years because of long-term estrogen use.

Estrogen Revisited: Lifelong and Fearless will ultimately provide the reader with a detailed explanation and summary of estrogen benefits and will illustrate a woman's physical aging process, the time span involved and options that may be available.

This book will also help men understand the feminine process of change with, and without, the usage of estrogen. Moreover, I encourage men to be active with their female partners to ensure that they have a complete understanding of the availability of alternate choices and the need for timely decisions. They can jointly discuss and participate in these major life choices. This book will also help men understand what happens when women approach the menopausal years and ways in which menopause affects their lives.

The book wholeheartedly disputes the WHI study results, as previously announced, and includes comprehensive charts and graphs with supporting data. The charts and graphs provide the reader with facts concerning breast cancer, coronary heart disease, hip fractures, Alzheimer's disease, dementia and premature mortality prevented in women taking estrogen.

My experience with estrogen, specifically Premarin, is the direct opposite of everything adversely published concerning estrogen. Hopefully, many of the other long-term estrogen users will contact me through my website (dwalters@menopausefree.org) and share their experiences as well. This information will create a database resulting in the first of its kind ever recorded. Already, women who have met me and know of my estrogen experience are amazed to learn of a completely different medical environment concerning estrogen.

I have written this book to bring awareness to four important aspects of the complicated estrogen environment: 1) long-term estrogen use, 2) excellent lifelong health well beyond the menopausal years, 3) never having to experience menopause and 4) women now have a choice.

My wish is that women worldwide will take the necessary action to become aware, informed and learn everything they can about their body's health, what changes will occur, when they will occur, and become active in decisions made relative to their health. The reward of this action can be good health well past the menopause age.

> "Estrogen therapy doesn't change a woman.
> On the contrary: it ***keeps her from changing.***"

> —Dr. Robert A. Wilson
>
> Feminine Forever, 1966

Blane Milton Crandall, M.D.

Why am I, Blane Milton Crandall, M.D., writing this book with Donna? I am not selling anything. I have already spent tens of thousands of dollars in advertisements and political contributions in an attempt to get someone to care about the inaccurate, incorrect conclusions of the Women's Health Initiative (WHI) study and what it is doing to women in this country and worldwide. It was my hope that academic and organized medicine would stop the madness that has resulted from that study, but they seem to be afraid. I am co-authoring this book with Donna concerning the important topic of estrogen use in an attempt to try to stop the ongoing disability; the taking of women's physical, mental, social, and emotional health; and the eventual premature death that will occur to millions of women in America and around the world. I have had a very successful obstetrical and gynecologic surgery practice, and this effort has consumed most of my spare time and most of my money over the last seven years. What I have that the WHI researchers do not have is over thirty years of experience prescribing estrogen and caring for women in offices, skilled nursing facilities, and hospitals.

This effort started when I began seeing and continued to see one to four women almost every day who had had their lives and health destroyed by either stopping or not starting postmenopausal estrogen replacement. Look at yourself; look at your loved ones who have stopped or not started estrogen. The rapid aging that occurs externally when estrogen levels decline also occurs internally. You and your physician have been mislead by epidemiologists, statisticians, and the news media into thinking that you are less likely to develop breast cancer if you do not take estrogen. They are lying! It is simply not true. Women who have never taken estrogen have just as much likelihood to develop breast cancer within one to two years as those who have, but those who have never taken estrogen have a worse chance of cure. I am not selling any hormones or lab tests. I am presenting the truth based on the excellent data of the WHI study and other studies which were incorrectly analyzed as a result of the authors having little or no understanding of the natural history of breast cancer, heart disease, or Alzheimer's disease; little or no experience in the prescribing of hormones; and little or no experience with the ongoing health care of women in skilled nursing facilities or hospitals.

My wife, Doshie, has been on estrogen for thirty-one years and will, with hope, continue on estrogen for another forty years or longer. She is years younger in appearance and health than women her age who did not start taking estrogen at menopause.

Read this book and save your life by demanding the hormones you deserve. Men, if you want your wife or loved one to grow old with you and not before you, encourage her to start or restart estrogen. Remember that during menopause, the brain starves and dies. Menopause is not osteoporosis, it is "body-porosis." During the week that I finished this book, two different women on the same day cried as I entered the exam room. I inquired as to what was wrong. The answer was the same from both: "Thank you for giving me my life back!" Do not let "them" take the life (health life, family life, marital life, business life, social life, or sex life) or health of you or your loved ones. If you are on hormones, continue taking them guilt free for the rest of your life. If you are in menopause and not on hormones, then start them now, no matter your age, and continue them for the rest of your life.

How, you may ask, can I say these things? I was trained in family practice from 1974 to 1977. I prescribed hormones and studied hormones from 1974 until now. I cared for women and men of all ages. I studied and treated heart disease, Alzheimer's disease, cerebrovascular disease, strokes, vascular dementia, fractures of all kinds, breast cancer, colon cancer, estrogen deficiency in women, and testosterone deficiency in men. I switched specialties in 1984, moving to obstetrics and gynecology, but I brought to my practice a unique understanding of other specialties. When I was invited to speakers' training with renowned hormone experts in early 2002, I heard of the web publication of the first WHI paper on estrogen and progestin. After reading this, I immediately realized that the authors had no apparent understanding of the natural history of heart disease, breast cancer, or stroke or any understanding of the pharmacology of the hormones they prescribed. I e-mailed the lead author and offered to come to the NIH at almost any time for almost any amount of time at my expense to help them understand their results. Unfortunately for the women of the world, I only received a condescending response both times I offered to come to the NIH and help them understand the real meaning of the excellent data they had accumulated. It is to be hoped that you, the reader, will be able to understand the real conclusions that should have been reached. I apologize in advance for lapsing into "medicalese" at times. We welcome questions, corrections, and debate. I have been told by leading academicians that the conclusions of the WHI "Are what they are" and will not be changed. The conclusions of the WHI and any paper that references the conclusions as fact are actually incorrect and nonsensical! I am willing to debate or discuss this at almost any time. The authors and academic gynecologists are apparently afraid of open debate. The sooner it is resolved, the sooner women will stop being afraid, injured, disabled, and killed.

The best mortality data available predicts that eight million women in the United States and about 100 million women worldwide will die prematurely over the next twenty-three years. These premature deaths are the direct responsibility of the WHI, NIH, FDA, and all other professional organizations that have failed to evaluate these studies scientifically, accepting the incorrect conclusions as fact.

You cannot acquire experience by making experiments. You cannot create experience. You must undergo it.

—Albert Camus (1913–1960)

Menopause...In the Beginning!

Donna Walters

Men-o-pause [F. ménopause, fr. méno-men-+pause, stop, pause] the period of natural cessation of menstruation occurring usually between the ages of forty-five and fifty. The word "meno+pause" comes from the Greek words for month and cessation.

According to modern medical history, the word menopause was first introduced around 1816 when French physician CPL de Gardarrne referred to this phase of a woman's life as *le ménespausie*. Over the past 500 years, menopause has been called many things, including the change of life, the climacteric, Indian summer, the time of life and the hormone deficiency disease. Medical diagnosis and records of menopause date back to the nineteenth century. Beyond that, we have only the letters and diaries of physicians to give us insight into menopause, its symptoms and treatment.

In Medieval Europe, the cessation of the "menses" was a cause for alarm; it was thought that women's sexual appetite increased dramatically even to the point of having demonic partners. A woman's breath was considered to be noxious, even toxic to children and pregnant women. In that period, there were few female physicians and female anatomy was a taboo subject because of religious and political beliefs. Therefore, little time or research was devoted to the subject.

When women reached menopausal years it was common practice to bleed a patient. This treatment was done by a phlebotomist; the objective being to rid the body of toxicity by bloodletting. Physicians also noticed that during the menstruation cessation, women developed all forms of diseases, including weakness, tumors, cancers and joint pain. Unfortunately, hormone replacement therapy was hundreds of years away. As a consequence, menopause remained virtually untreated well into the twentieth century.

In 1929, the first American doctors to treat menopause were E.L. Severinghaus and J. Evans. The treatment they used was a derivative from the amniotic fluid of cattle. In 1930, Dr. Bernhard Zondek discovered that pregnant mares urine contained water-soluble estrogens. By 1933, a product made from the urine of pregnant women, Emmenin, became the first estrogen replacement product marketed in the United States. In 1942, Premarin, was introduced into the marketplace and by 1960, estrogen replacement therapy was used by twelve percent of all menopausal women and became the number one drug of choice for treating menopausal symptoms.

There are three stages of menopause:

1. **Perimenopause** is the early stage of menopause during which the hormone levels are affected. The age when perimenopause begins varies, but it may begin as early as age thirty-five and can last up to six years.

2. **Menopause** is when the ovaries stop producing the estrogen hormone, ending both the menstrual period and the fertility process. Natural menopause occurs for most women between the ages of forty-five and fifty-five and can take anywhere from five to ten years from the starting point until the process is completed.

3. **Postmenopause** is the time period after the actual menopause process is completed.

Seemingly between early puberty, PMS, perimenopause, menopause and the post-menopause depression, we are doomed to emotional stress. Can we be more up and down??? I'm hot. I'm cold. I'm pissed off. I'm sad. I'm pissed off again! Our poor husbands. Having their trusty Viagra matters not! We're just not in the mood. It's simply a wonder we last through long-term marriages.

Symptoms

The following are some symptoms that may be associated with menopause and estrogen deficiency:

- ♀ Hot flashes, night sweats, extreme sweating, temperature changes
- ♀ Headaches, migraines, frequent urination
- ♀ Achy joints
- ♀ Weak bones
- ♀ Difficulty in falling asleep
- ♀ Insomnia, early wakening
- ♀ Day-long fatigue, reduced stamina
- ♀ Depression, minor anxiety
- ♀ Problems with short-term memory or difficulty in concentrating
- ♀ Mood changes
- ♀ Lessened interest in self-image and appearance
- ♀ Decreased sense of sexuality
- ♀ Dry skin and eyes, loss of skin radiance
- ♀ Changes in sexual desire, pain during sexual activity
- ♀ Vaginal dryness
- ♀ Loss of fullness of the breasts
- ♀ Thinning hair
- ♀ Weight gain and sensations of bloating

Estrogen, Menopause & Aging

The following are major topics and concerns of women:

- ♀ Women are always interested in issues concerning their *health*.
- ♀ Women are interested in products that will help maintain their *youth*.
- ♀ Women are interested in issues concerning *weight control*.
- ♀ Women are interested in their *sexuality*.
- ♀ Women do not welcome *menopause* or growing old.
- ♀ The Women's Health Initiative (WHI) study of 2002 created an enormous amount of fear and confusion for women concerning *estrogen use* — this apprehension still exists today. That fear, however, is unfounded.

All of the above topics are directly related to estrogen, menopause and aging. A woman's body and health *require* estrogen. What hasn't been made clear in the past is — *how are they all connected to each other?*

NO MORE MENOPAUSE!   PERIOD.

There are more than 6.3 million estrogen users, and I want each and every one of them to feel supported in her choice.

As a result of the seven-year state of fear and confusion that has continued to plague women due to the WHI study, I am doing something that has never been done before. I am going public with the story of my experience, and more importantly, the story of two medical situations that have never been publicized, discussed or acknowledged: *successful long-term estrogen use* and *never having menopause*! These two issues have never received publicity and yet millions of women have experienced both. The results of both long-term estrogen use and not experiencing menopause will increase a woman's experience of sustaining good health and vitality well past her menopausal years. *The time has arrived to tell the complete estrogen story* and to challenge the WHI study results and expose the harm created in its aftermath.

Medical studies are great when used as an informational tool. However, keep in mind that some studies do not always include certain aspects of their research. For example, data regarding age, hereditary factors and lifestyle preferences can change the results of any study. In the case of the '02 WHI study, you would think that an issue concerning something as important as women's lifelong health, and the ability to see and ask questions of women who have actually *experienced* long-term estrogen use, would be extremely advantageous. I am bringing attention to the fact that those studies were being conducted on only one-half of the problem — menopausal women who take hormone replacement treatments for the short-term and who are at an older age. What does the other side of estrogen use reveal? What about long-term estrogen users and/or those women who started taking it at a younger age? How can there be a complete picture or an accurate result without both sides being studied and researched?

It's been many years since that initial, half-truth study from the WHI was publicized and now we're finding several new answers from recent scientific studies. For example, announced in August 2009, a groundbreaking study revealed that certain kinds of hormone replacement therapy have now been proven to help prevent breast cancer in younger women. Prevent? Yes, according to NaturalNews.com a research team, consisting of scientists from several parts of the world, has discovered that a full complement of the sex hormones (estrogen, progesterone and testosterone) and their receptors is what helps to prevent breast cancer. It provides a reason why we don't see breast cancer in young, teenage girls — a time when all of the hormones are at optimum levels. This study shows that there is a very good reason why breast cancer does not appear until women reach the age of hormone imbalance and decline.

Another recent study from Italian scientists concludes that estrogen can kill mesothelioma cells. Statistically, women often have less aggressive mesothelioma tumors and survive longer than men. They had hypothesized that the hormone estrogen and estrogen receptors may be involved and according to the Surviving Mesothelioma website, they were right.

During a lecture given in 2009, Dr. Leon Speroff, a national expert in the field of reproductive endocrinology and professor of obstetrics and gynecology, said the benefits of hormonal treatment are numerous, from preventing fractures and osteoporosis, to likely reducing the risk of colorectal and ovarian cancer.

Yesterday, most women viewed estrogen as harmful and dangerous. Hopefully today, after reading this book and becoming familiar with the total estrogen environment, it will be viewed, at the very least, as user friendly.

YOU DON'T HAVE TO CHOOSE NATURAL DECAY
AND ATROPHY.
YOU CAN ALWAYS CHOOSE TO *NEVER*
HAVE MENOPAUSE.

Did You Know?

The following thought-provoking questions might be of interest:

Did you know that if a woman maintains her estrogen, she will not have menopause?

Did you know that the total risk of dying while taking hormones decreased by thirty-seven percent as revealed in an eighteen-year study, and the Kaiser Permanente twenty-three-year mortality study shows a thirty-three percent decrease?

Did you know estrogen protects a woman's coronary arteries and once the estrogen is depleted, she loses that protection? Data and statistics state that heart disease is the number one cause of death among women.

Did you know that if a woman has to undergo any type of heart surgery, the instruments used are those which are fitted to a man? Those improperly sized instruments could increase women's risks for other serious ailments.

Did you know that if you contract breast cancer, and are taking estrogen, you will have a less severe case of breast cancer?

Did you know that women taking hormones have a twenty percent **decrease** risk of dying from breast cancer?

Did you know that being overweight or obese increases the risk of breast cancer especially if a woman is past menopause and/or if they gained the weight later in life?

Did you know a woman's chance of being diagnosed with breast cancer increases with age? When a woman is in her thirties, her chances are one in two hundred thirty-three and by the time she is in her eighties, that risk is one in eight?

Did you know heart disease is the number one cause of death for women with more than 246,000 deaths each year? The second most common cause of death is stroke (96,000 cases). The third cause of death is lung cancer (71,000 cases). The fourth cause of death is lower respiratory diseases (67,000 cases) and the fifth cause of death is breast cancer (40,000 cases).

Did you know there is compelling evidence that estrogen is necessary for glucose to cross the blood brain barrier? Without glucose the brain dies. A hot flash is the brain screaming out for glucose. When the hot flashes stop, that part of the brain has died.

Did you know that seventy-one percent of nursing home patients are women? Two out of three probably would not be there if they had been on hormones.

Did you know weight gain can be a result of menopause? The endocrine system of women, because of their hormone balance, makes it difficult for them to lose weight after the age of 40. Weight gain for women is governed by two groups of hormones, sex hormones (estrogen) and thyroid hormones. Womanly figures are a result of estrogens, which form their busts, thighs, stomach, buttocks, slims the waist, softens the skin and helps to decrease a woman's appetite. Equally important is the DHEA hormone, which also decreases after age forty. Again, another negative result of menopause.

Did you know that women who are not taking hormones have four times as much Alzheimer's disease as men?

Did you know hip fractures are twice as common in women not taking hormones? Fifteen percent of women with hip fractures will be dead in six months. Twenty-five percent will never walk independently again. Estrogen is twice as effective as other therapies in preventing osteoporosis.

Did you know there are more than 6.3 million women taking estrogen? The Food and Drug Administration (FDA) has implemented the guidelines for estrogen use to be limited to the lowest dosage for the shortest period of time. However, they overlooked one specific group of estrogen users — the millions of women who have taken it for more than twenty-plus years. One woman, who lives in the Washington, DC area, is ninety-four years old and has been taking estrogen for fifty-three years. Look at the hardship those guidelines have placed on the millions of long-term estrogen users — the group that has never been acknowledged or included in studies. Who is going to fix that catastrophe — and when?

Did you know that more than 458 million women have taken oral contraceptives and that they contain estrogen? Did you ever think about how long women have taken birth control pills — maybe as long as twenty, thirty or even forty years?

IT'S YOUR CHOICE.

1. Menopause is *not* a necessary part of a woman's life and could actually be medically harmful for some women.

2. Given today's medical capabilities and the fact that the average life expectancy for women is eighty years, menopause should be an elective process. Women should be given the opportunity to make the decision of whether menopause is something they want to experience during their lifetime.

3. The FDA needs to change its latest recommendations concerning the use of estrogen by making separate guidelines for the various uses of estrogen rather than categorizing estrogen use for only menopausal symptoms.

4. Studies and research need to include information and statistics from the millions of women who have taken estrogen for longer than

twenty years. Even if this information is from an observational standpoint, its impact will create a more balanced estrogen environment to help women know the outcome of long-term estrogen users.

Since the medical establishment is far behind the times concerning either the improvement or elimination of menopause, it's time to give women the information and let them make the choice — just like women did when the birth control pill came out sixty years ago. As Dr. Crandall says…

DEMAND YOUR HORMONES!

The Estrogen Challenge

I have been taking estrogen for more than thirty years. As a result of the WHI study, the Food and Drug Administration (FDA) has decided that estrogen should be taken for the shortest recommended time and at the lowest recommended dosage. However, in making those recommendations, they overlooked the millions of long-term estrogen users who have been taking it for more than twenty years, most of whom were without incident. The issue is that they did not establish separate guidelines for the various uses of estrogen. There are four different groups (see page 70) of estrogen users, but the guidelines established are only for the menopausal women. As a result, the estrogen environment has become dangerous for all estrogen users.

I challenge the Women's Health Initiative's view on estrogen, menopause and aging. With detailed examples of a woman's life — my life — and the health advantages experienced as a result of maintaining estrogen life-long and *without* experiencing menopause, I hope to dispel the misleading results of the WHI studies. My co-author, Blane Crandall, M.D., concurs with my stance. In several chapters he includes detailed explanations of hormone replacement therapy as it relates to the different estrogen users. Further, Dr. Crandall provides undisputed evidence that reveals the incorrect conclusions of the WHI study.

The estrogen environment is complicated. There are many books available concerning menopause and estrogen and the recommendations in those books vary from one extreme to another. *Estrogen Revisited: Lifelong and Fearless* is not a typical book dealing with the subject of menopause or suggestions of how to cope with menopause. Rather, it is the direct opposite: it tells of life *without* menopause and it is not your mother's estrogen book of the 1960s.

An important part missing from the estrogen environment is the stories of millions of women who can share their experiences and answer questions of long-term estrogen use. The participants of most of the studies are older women, and the studies are usually conducted for short periods of time. There are more than three million long-term estrogen users. It only seems logical that their estrogen experiences would be as valuable as, or more so than, the inconclusive study results that have been furnished thus far. Just imagine the medical information that would be available today if data had been obtained (clinical or observational) from this unique set of long-term estrogen users.

COULD LONG-TERM ESTROGEN REPLACEMENT BE RIGHT FOR YOU?

Ask yourself these questions:

1. Do you want *only* fifty years of good health before deterioration sets in?

2. Do you want to maintain your femininity throughout your life or experience its loss once your estrogen supply is depleted?

3. Do you want to increase your chances for heart disease—the number one cause of death for women—because the estrogen that provides protection to your coronary arteries is gone?

4. Do you want to risk hip fractures and other diseases because of estrogen deficiency?

5. Why should women lose their health (which is a result of menopause) because their body stops producing estrogen?

The time is now for women to know exactly what their health needs are and what they will be in the future. This information will enable them to begin a preventative treatment plan *well in advance* of any deterioration of their health. Any action taken must begin **before** menopause or the onset of the aging process.

Today, more than ever before, women are obtaining college degrees, including advanced degrees and PhDs. They sit on the boards of major corporations; they are doctors, lawyers, teachers, members of Congress, and Supreme Court justices. For many years, the Secretary of State has been a woman, and for the first time in history, the Speaker of the House of Representatives for the 110th Congress, first session, is a woman. Recently, a woman ran for president, the highest office in the United States. Most of these women accomplished their goals after the age of fifty. Women have attained success in important job positions and raised families, too. The glass ceiling may not be broken yet, but there is a huge crack.

With all the accomplishments of women worldwide over the past century, why must we accept token or fallacious medical advice concerning estrogen and menopause that is based on inconclusive or flawed data from a government-sponsored study? Why must women endure menopause, which is a chemical change that takes away their health and womanhood when they have many productive years left? Why should we invite the withering process when there is a viable alternative? Medical science has made important strides in treating and curing diseases in the past twenty years. Many new and exciting drugs have come into the marketplace to help physicians treat illnesses and diseases; however, digressive studies and a laissez faire attitude in the medical community have maintained, rather than improved, the treatment for menopause. Continuance of this attitude is unconscionable. The medical community has allowed this position to be today's acceptable medical environment for women. Are these the best medical advancements that can be provided to women in the twenty-first century?

Menopause can be a devastating health problem for some women. Hence, the time has arrived for the medical community to present women with accurate information rather than inconclusive results from patchwork studies that have not been independently verified. I am here to reveal the advantages that long-term estrogen use has and its effect on a woman's total health in areas such as cardiovascular, bones, skin, eyes, mental state of mind, sexuality factors, energy levels and the aging process, just to name a few. Further, I am giving you a realistic example of estrogen awareness and have recorded it in a manner of experience — *not controversial and inaccurate studies!*

With knowledge of the entire estrogen environment, women, together with their physician, should be able to make an informed decision relative to their specific health needs and requirement.

<u>Doing Nothing vs. Taking Action</u>

Only two options are available for dealing with menopause: (1) doing nothing and allowing the natural process to take its course, or (2) taking hormone replacement therapy. The problem with the latter choice is that women basically rely on someone else's professional advice without knowing in advance what the results will be after taking hormone replacement therapy. Isn't that true of many new drugs? We don't even know the long-term effects of using cell phones. We take those kinds of risks daily. It's our prerogative. There are many websites and printed materials on both choices concerning HRT, but a woman ultimately has to make the decision and hope her choice is correct and will benefit her health. A fully informed decision today, because it is based upon the incomplete information and results of research and scientific studies presently available, is almost impossible to make.

There are numerous menopause organizations and affiliates whose mission is to help provide support and give information to women as they go through the menopause process. I spoke with the founder and president of one such organization, and in her view, women were not interested in learning about menopause. She came to this conclusion based on the lack of attendance of women at seminars held to furnish information. Women know, however, there is nothing favorable any organization can offer, be it information or advice, which will allow avoidance of menopause or make the whole process easier to endure. If those same organizations could offer hope for the future in terms of alleviating menopause or at the very least making the process less severe, women would be very interested in what these organizations had to say. Yet, to date, nothing has ever improved or changed.

I spoke with two women in my office who recently experienced the menopause process, and their descriptions were tales of horror. One of the women said, "You wake up one day and know that you are old. You look, feel and know you now old, and there is nothing that you can do to change it. Your womanly instincts are gone and you just don't care in the same manner that you had for an entire lifetime. There is nothing you can do but accept it. Your attitude toward your marriage, your family and children, and your job is an attitude of just not caring — you really just don't care anymore! The agonizing health changes are drastic, and when you have passed through the menopause process, you know that you are no longer the same person you had been for over fifty years. I never knew menopause would be this bad."

<u>The Truth of the Matter</u>

The real truth of the matter is that menopause is the premature advancement into old age. Every seven minutes, one of us will turn fifty. That means that within the time it takes you to shower, blow dry what's left of your hair and pluck the one on your chin, five more women will be looking at the maturing reflection in their mirrors and asking themselves, "Good God, when did that happen?" There are thirty-eight million baby boomer women pioneering their way through this new version of growing old. We are in uncharted territory. And thanks to modern science, twenty more years have been added to our lifespan.

Menopause in women has no counterpart in men of similar age. In 1890, the average life expectancy of women was forty-two. In 1910, the average life expectancy increased to be about 50. Many women in the 1900's did not live past fifty so many did not experience menopause. Today, however, old age is now re-defined as the late 70's and 80's putting women living twenty to thirty years past the menopause age of fifty-one.

Once the menopause process (which can last up to ten years) has been completed, most women will have lost their good health and energy. They will appear haggard and wrinkled, their breasts will sag, and their sexual desires will diminish. This is a very general description of the result of menopause. Please note that many of these drastic changes and loss of womanhood may become ***permanent*** if not reversed by HRT which may be taken at any age, even in the eighties and nineties.

What Purpose Does Menopause Serve?

In Search of the Answer

As a direct result of my specific situation, I have yet to find anyone able to answer a very important question: What purpose does menopause serve? In other words, is the actual natural process something that improves the quality of a woman's life or is it detrimental to a woman's overall wellbeing? I ask such a question because medically speaking, no one has been able to provide an answer other than by stating, "It is a process every woman must endure." My response to that statement is, "Why?" One person whom I spoke with at the National Menopause Organization answered the question by saying, "It's nature's way." I have great difficulty with that response. It's also nature's way to contract meningitis, polio, ear infections and mumps. Should women today — in this age of unprecedented and life-altering medical advancements — have to experience the upsetting process of ending their womanhood?

The medical environment is too advanced *not* to be able to find a way in which to circumvent the negative results of the lengthy menopause process. I believe the exposure of my particular situation will benefit women a great deal and will, with hope, be a catalyst to changing the thinking about the entire menopause process. I have known and enjoyed my youthful sexuality for my entire life. I cannot imagine life any other way. I recently purchased a hormone level test at my local grocery store. The test registered a normal hormone result, but then that is a result of taking estrogen for almost 30 years. Can you imagine being 62 years old and having a normal hormone level?

We Need More Now!

I think my life experiences, as well as those of other women who have taken estrogen for the long-term, should show the scientists, the researchers, and the medical and pharmaceutical industries that more studies and/or additional drugs are needed. Researchers should focus on helping women achieve a pleasant life, similar to mine, as they reach their late forties and fifties so that they do not experience the worry or burden of a ten-year, demoralizing menopause experience. Waiting until women reach the age of fifty to treat menopause is waiting too long. My belief: Research and studies are missing the target. When a woman reaches her fifties, any medical changes she will experience may have started or have already taken place and may be irreversible by that time. To receive the optimum benefits of any medical condition, corrective actions need to be implemented *before* changes occur.

I recently met a woman flight attendant who told me that her mother had a rough encounter with menopause and was completely through the process by age forty-two. As a result, the flight attendant's own physician put her on a low dosage of birth control pills fourteen years ago to help her maintain her estrogen level, and she has yet to have one symptom of menopause though she is in her fifties. She, too, based on her experience, believes that there is great merit in the theory of maintaining the estrogen level throughout a woman's later years. How many more women are there with similar positive life experiences who can help to confirm the benefits of continued, long-term estrogen use?

Additional Keys to Success

There are other important factors that contribute to my good health, including diet, exercise, mental attitude, and the fact that I have used Retin A on my face for almost twenty years. Even though all of those factors have been important during my lifetime, the most important aspect is that I have been, and continue to be, a very happy woman and have always lived my life with a positive outlook regardless of the many obstacles encountered. I do not know how I would have felt if I had to suffer through the agonizing and difficult menopause process. If that had been the case, I am fairly sure that my happiness would have dissipated over those sixty years.

Dr. Crandall Gives Us Some Answers

The answers to many of Donna's questions are known. However, they have not been answered with forty-year double blind, placebo-controlled studies. Using a control or placebo group would withhold estrogen from women that would put them at unacceptable risk. Risk of osteoporosis, heart attack, Alzheimer's, sexual dysfunction and premature death would all be increased. This is why thyroid hormone, insulin, and cortisone replacement have never been studied with double blind, placebo-controlled studies. Giving a placebo instead of real thyroid hormone, insulin or cortisone in a blinded study is illogical and dangerous. Estrogen deficiency is just as dangerous and devastating as these other hormone deficiencies — it just happens slower. The decision to use insulin, thyroid replacement and cortisone replacement was based on observation and the historical consequences of not taking them. Physicians, patients, friends, and family observe the consequences of not using estrogen in menopause. Excellent large observational studies confirm the findings of clinicians and family when women receive estrogen or when they do not receive estrogen. In summary:

1. Estrogen replacement should begin when the uterus and ovaries are removed in a pre-menopausal woman and should continue for life.

2. Estrogen and cycled or continuous progestin or progesterone should be started at the time of removal of both ovaries in pre-menopausal women. The progestin or progesterone protects the uterus from endometrial cancer. This should be continued for life.

3. At menopause, estrogen and cycled or continuous progestin or progesterone should be started and continued for life in a woman who has not had a hysterectomy.

4. A young woman who has had a hysterectomy without removal of the ovaries should start estrogen at menopause (when the ovaries stop working) and continue it for life.

These recommendations do not agree with the Women's Health Initiative (WHI)[2,3] because the WHI is wrong! The conclusions of the WHI were made with no apparent understanding of the natural history of the diseases discussed, the healthcare of women, or the pharmacology of the hormones used. The WHI study will be reviewed in this book at length, along with other studies, to help the reader reach his or her own conclusions.

Estrogen should be taken to alleviate estrogen deficiency. Progesterone or progestin is given to prevent endometrial cancer. These hormones should not be assumed to treat any other disease. Women who are estrogen deficient and do *not* take estrogen have a higher risk of heart attack,[4] fractures,[4] loss of height and spinal deformity, Alzheimer's disease,[4,5,6] death from breast cancer,[7] developing and dying from colon cancer, and loss of independence. Estrogen replacement is very similar to thyroid hormone replacement. If someone with thyroid deficiency does not take a thyroid hormone replacement, he or she will frequently eventually develop muscle edema and congestive heart failure. No physician would ever suggest prescribing a thyroid hormone replacement to treat congestive heart failure. Physicians would replace the thyroid and treat the heart with heart medications. Women should take estrogen and enjoy the benefits, but they should try to prevent and treat other diseases and deficiencies appropriately.

Donna is living proof of the benefits of lifelong estrogen use. Her case is not unique. She feels unique, however, because her physicians have been trying to take her off hormones since the WHI estrogen and progestin study[2] was published in July of 2002. In addition, women are afraid to say they are on estrogen or hormones because they are tired of listening to people telling them to stop taking hormones.

Physicians tried to stop Donna from taking Premarin because they either believed the conclusions of the WHI study or they were afraid of legal action that could be taken if she develops breast cancer or has a heart attack. Breast cancer is the most common kind of cancer in nonsmoking women[8], and heart attack is the leading cause of death in women[9] whether or not hormones are used. The risk of developing these problems is unfortunately not decreased if Donna stops taking Premarin. Once again I must state that the conclusions and the recommendations of the WHI are wrong! Expert committees of several professional organizations allegedly reviewed the study and agreed. Critical reviews were not performed, however; only comment and placid agreement with the conclusions resulted. Critical review with careful reading and an understanding of the natural history of breast cancer,[10,11] heart attack,[12] stroke, and thrombotic disease and the pharmacology of Premarin and oral progestin[13] leads to the following correct conclusions:

1. All the breast cancer was present when the study started. It was found earlier in the women taking conjugated equine estrogen (Premarin or CEE) plus medroxyprogesterone acetate (MPA) after the fourth year. There was no new breast cancer!

2. Taking oral CEE plus MPA precipitates heart attacks that were ready to happen. Women taking a placebo had just as many heart attacks within one year. Heart attacks develop fifteen to twenty years after a cholesterol plaque forms.

3. Strokes that were ready to happen were brought on after two to four years by taking oral CEE plus MPA. Women on no hormones had just as many strokes within one year.

4. The risk of hip fracture rises slowly at first but after five years begins to rise rapidly in the placebo group, while the risk of fracture in the CEE plus MPA group has almost stopped rising.

5. The only statistically significant results were more blood clots in the legs and fewer other osteoporotic fractures (not hip or spine) in the women taking oral CEE plus MPA.

6. Most of the women had pre-existing conditions, such as smoking, prior smoking, high cholesterol, hypertension, diabetes, heart attack, angina, prior blood clots in the legs or lungs, and prior stroke. These existing conditions are relative reasons not to take oral hormones.

7. Dosing was the same for all women. No physician would start insulin or thyroid hormone therapy at estimated full-replacement levels. The side effects and risks would be too great. Many women received too much or too little hormone. Most should have been given a different estrogen by a different delivery system, such as a patch or gel.

8. The correct conclusions are that giving estrogen and progestin in the wrong amount and by the wrong route to the wrong women causes little harm or benefit over 5.6 years. The rapid rise in hip fractures in the placebo group as the study was ending, as well as the decrease in colon cancer in the CEE plus MPA group, would have quickly become significant if the study had not been hysterically stopped.

Attention — Improvement — Advancement

Donna Walters

I thought my situation was somewhat unusual, but since working alongside Dr. Crandall while writing this book, I have found evidence of many women taking estrogen for lengthy periods of time with good results and without side effects. How did the industry come to base their trials and studies on women who were way past the beginning stages of menopause? Apparently, everyone was, and continues to be, only interested in helping to alleviate the symptoms without ever giving serious thought to changing the menopause process. The target has been missed, and women have been the recipients of bad decisions made on their behalf by the government, the pharmaceutical industry, and the medical profession.

A form of communication should be established so there can be input and feedback from women who have had similar experiences or who also may have lived their lives without enduring the menopause process. Such data would be very important in establishing factual and complete information concerning the estrogen environment.

Creating extreme attention, as well as a concerted effort, in an attempt to help women achieve a lifetime of good health is absolutely vital. By today's standards, on average, the first fifty years of a woman's life are good and productive, but the years that follow begin to deteriorate and ultimately could be considered sub-standard. Women should voice their concern loudly about only having good health for about half of their lives while advocating the decline of good health after menopause as unacceptable.

Note: I am not supporting, confirming, or denying any theories or medical statements. I am only bringing an awareness of the whole complicated estrogen environment to the attention of women rather than just bits and pieces.

Awareness Factor #1

If women can be prescribed estrogen for more than twenty years without negative consequences, then it's time for confirmation and recognition of its benefits.

Awareness Factor #2

It is inexcusable that the only relatively current studies are incomplete and based on a distinct class of menopausal and post-menopausal women. How did the people performing research miss such an important group of cases involving women who had been taking estrogen for longer than twenty years?

Awareness Factor #3

The entire medical industry knows estrogen replacement is required in two particular situations: 1) women who have undergone hysterectomies at an early age; and 2) women exhibiting pre-menopausal symptoms. Yet, there is no protocol in place for the length of time estrogen should be used after a woman experiences a hysterectomy at an early age.

Maybe if women voice their views and concerns, such protests will help gain the attention of the medical community and place a higher importance level on menopause with the goal of seeking more research and funding. Perhaps now is the time that everyone involved with menopause (physicians, researchers, scientists, and pharmaceutical companies) should go beyond the accepted treatment (which is to prescribe hormones for a few years to ease the symptoms) and perform more in-depth studies as to the cause.

In the late 1960s, my father-in-law had serious heart disease and was asked by National Institutes of Health to be a patient for a new and radical procedure called heart bypass surgery. His family was shocked at such a radical idea and declined. However, such a treatment, with improvement and development over time, became commonplace in the medical community and has saved many lives. What radical ideas have ever emerged concerning menopause? I try to understand in today's world, in which medical technology continues to rapidly advance in many areas, why the treatment of menopause is as archaic as decades past? What message does that send to women concerning the importance of menopause and, to a greater degree, women's health issues? Why are we deemed as disposable and useless by a male-dominated practice, upon reaching a mature age?

Dr. Crandall

In order to further illustrate the complexity of the estrogen environment, listed below are many positive results of estrogen use. How many of the items listed below have you learned about?

1. A new study has found that women who have their ovaries removed (which stops estrogen production) increase their chances of coronary heart disease, stroke, breast cancer, ovarian cancer, lung cancer, colorectal cancer, total cancers, hip fracture, pulmonary embolus, and death from all causes.

2. Hormones produced by the ovaries keep the heart, bones and blood vessels healthy.

3. Data analyzed on 2,050 people between 1997 and 2004 have indicated that there is growing evidence that estrogen protects against colorectal cancer.

4. Research indicates that women taking postmenopausal hormone therapy reduced the risk for colorectal cancer by about 40%.

5. There is a study that revealed that estrogen deficiency causes bladder hypersensitity.

6. Estrogen users perform better on memory tests than non-users.

7. Studies are being conducted because evidence indicates that estrogen may prevent Alzheimer's disease.

8. Research indicates that estrogen promises new hope to both men and women who suffer from the symptoms of schizophrenia.

9. A study revealed that estrogen therapy seems to protect against brain damage for women in their late 40s and 50s.

10. There is evidence that hormone therapy may help protect older women against age related blindness.

11. A study published in the *Journal of the American Medical Association*, stated that men with heart failure who had the lowest levels of estrogen had about four times the risk of dying as men with average levels.

12. A recent study revealed that estrogen strengthens women's immune systems.

13. Estrogen therapy can help control metastatic breast cancer as reported by the results of a study through the National Cancer Institute. "About 40,000 women die of metastatic breast cancer each year, and estrogen therapy potentially could help thousands of women with hormone receptor-positive disease," says Matthew Ellis, M.B., Ph.D., associate professor of medicine at Washington University School of Medicine in St. Louis.

14. Dr. Delfin Tan, International Menopause Society board member, states, "Estrogen affects many target organs through a variety of estrogen receptors in diverse tissues." Further, he states, "This causes changes in the brain, eyes, heart, breast, vasomotor system, colon and urogenital tract." Also, Dr. Tan lists osteoporosis, atherosclerosis, coronary heart disease, cerebrovascular disease, and Alzheimer's disease as the late effects of estrogen deficiency.

The Society of Obstetricians and Gynaecologists of Canada (SOGC) Update

It gives me great pleasure to share with you the following public information as recently disclosed by the Society of Obstetricians and Gynaecologists of Canada (SOGC) who has challenged the notion that hormone therapy does more harm than good. They have a position paper with their findings as described by a panel of Canada's top experts in women's health and menopause. (See www.medicalnewstoday.com/articles/136655.php)

Their findings, as outlined in the above referenced document, bring attention to important facts that all women need to know. For example:

1. There is a definite need to get the real facts in order to provide quality advice to women and their health-care providers.

2. Misunderstandings as a result of the early analysis and reporting of the Women's Health Initiative (WHI) research results as announced in 2002 must be addressed.

3. The WHI study created fear among women that short-term estrogen use will increase the chances of getting breast cancer. That concern is unfounded.

4. Disperse new information concerning osteoporosis risk, and the effect menopause can have on cardiovascular disease and cognitive function.

5. Share their finding by a panel that HT does not increase the risk of heart attack in younger women experiencing menopause.

6. The importance of the timing of estrogen use relative to risks for breast cancer, heart disease and cognitive decline.

7. The Update confirmed that "one in two women over 50 will suffer an osteoporosis-related fracture in their remaining lifetime, which can cause chronic pain, reduced mobility, loss of independence, and increased risk of death."

The Forgotten Few

Donna Walters

Expose the Unknown

There is a group of three million women who have been taking estrogen long-term for more than twenty years. I refer to this special, unique group of women of long-term estrogen use as the "Forgotten Few." What is difficult to understand concerning this group is the fact that they were prescribed estrogen exclusively when the medical industry had no advance knowledge or medical evidence as to what the result would be for them after an extended period of time.

Historically speaking, estrogen was approved and placed in the market in 1942. Sixty-seven years have passed and its risks and benefits are still unknown. The absence of this important knowledge prevents women from feeling secure about what action they should take regarding its use and the duration of treatment. All of the previous studies concerning estrogen were associated with the *prevention* of different *diseases*, such as heart disease, breast cancer, blood clots, colon cancer, osteoporosis, bone fractures, dementia, and Alzheimer's disease, and the general quality of life regarding energy levels, sleep, and sexual activity. No studies have been conducted, or are ongoing, to determine whether estrogen could be used within the menopause environment to *prevent* menopause and its accompanying symptoms. Also, there have been no studies or related research performed in order to determine what the result would be if estrogen was supplemented so that a woman's body did not undergo a complete depletion of estrogen during her life.

My decision to remain on estrogen alone was based on experiencing a lifetime of excellent health, not on any medical fact or evidence relating thereto because neither exists to this day. For whatever reason, the group of women receiving estrogen alone, and their specific cases, are not mentioned or publicized. Hopefully, exposing my specific case will help to emphasize the need to apply pressure to the medical industry. Members of the industry must be persuaded to include, consider, and protect the concerns of *all women* relative to estrogen use and not just those in a specific age group, those in a specific medical area, or those suffering from a specific disease.

<u>Confused, Concerned but Not Undecided</u>

I am sure the Forgotten Few are equally concerned and probably even more confused now that the NIH and FDA have deemed it appropriate to change the prescription guidelines regarding the usage of estrogen. My difficult decision to remain on the same dosage and prescription was based on the following three very important reasons:

1. **<u>EXCELLENT HEALTH</u>**. I have experienced a lifetime, more than sixty years, of excellent health.

2. **<u>SAFE REGIMEN.</u>** I do not know what result I would experience if I stopped taking estrogen. Without any knowledge or medical evidence based on studies regarding the Forgotten Few to furnish that important answer, I feel that it would be medically safer to continue the same regimen that I have maintained for the past thirty years.

3. **<u>EMBRACING EXPERIENCE</u>.** I personally do not believe the deteriorating health (or side effects) as a result of menopause should be part of a woman's life, especially given today's standard of living and general medical advances. I have never

experienced menopause, have had excellent health without it, and do not want my lifestyle changed in any manner, especially as I approach the senior citizen age group.

My Life Without Menopause

Calculated Conclusion

As a result of not being part of a case study, or knowing anyone else with the similar characteristics, and because there has been no medical data collected or recorded on me or anyone with similar characteristics, everything stated herein is a calculated conclusion and opinion made without medical study or related documentation.

Frozen in Time

I am actually embarrassed to admit that until recently I had no knowledge of the menopause process even though my mother underwent a complete hysterectomy at age twenty-four and I, too, underwent a hysterectomy (including ovaries) at age thirty-one. My physician prescribed estrogen (Premarin) immediately following the surgery, and almost thirty years later, I am still taking Premarin. Medically speaking, my menopause occurred at the time of the hysterectomy (surgical menopause), although no symptoms were evident because I was taking estrogen. My medical state of being and everything associated with me was seemingly frozen in time at the age Premarin was first ingested.

Recently, a telephone call was placed to the National Council on Aging to ask questions relative to estrogen. Upon informing the person I was speaking to of how long I had been taking estrogen, interesting advice was received, albeit off the record. Scientists, I was told, believe the secret to the success of estrogen is based upon the age at which a woman commences usage. In other words, if a person begins taking estrogen *before* her body starts the menopause process, she will have a much higher success rate, because there will be no lapse in hormone production and menopause will be prevented from ever occurring.

Estrogen and the Heart

The medical industry wants to know if estrogen plays an important role in preventing cardiovascular disease. Indeed, in many of the books and articles that I have read, including some of the studies from clinical trials, the area of cardiovascular disease has been an important area of interest. Again, my situation in the area of cardiovascular disease is probably unlike any other that has been medically recorded, and all I can do is report what has happened to me — and how it relates to my specific situation.

When I was in my late thirties, my doctor diagnosed me with high cholesterol with my level being in the mid to high three hundreds. I was put on cholesterol-lowering medication approximately twenty years ago (before they had statins), and the dosage has, over the years, increased to where it is now — the maximum dosage of eighty milligrams a day. My cholesterol readings have varied, and last year, my cholesterol level reached almost five hundred, with my triglyceride level reaching almost eight hundred. Please keep in mind: The average level of cholesterol should be two hundred or below and the triglyceride level should be approximately one hundred and fifty. As a result of my history of high cholesterol, approximately ten years ago, my cardiologist scheduled me to undergo an angiogram. The results showed my arteries to be wide open with no signs of any cardiovascular disease. **He advised me at that time that the estrogen I had been on for many years had protected my arteries.**

Interesting to note, I have had almost thirty years of extremely high cholesterol levels and have not experienced any cardiovascular disease. I wish I could say that result was due to taking statins, but the truth is my cholesterol levels were extremely high for many years prior to taking medication. Is there any way estrogen contributed to keeping my arteries open and free from any calcification? Does my example indicate favorable benefits to cardiovascular health from long-term estrogen use? Again, there is no current information that can be used to answer this question, only my personal experience and comment from my doctor.

The following items are brief descriptions of major medical areas relative to my specific health:

1. **Cholesterol**. As noted, I have had extremely high cholesterol levels since my thirties and have been on cholesterol-lowering medicine for almost twenty-five years. However, with medication, my cholesterol level is presently 188, my HDL level is 73, and my LDL level is 63. I recently had a thallium stress test that revealed my heart was functioning at a 72 percent level although the average rate for my age group is 40 percent to 50 percent. I have also had a C-protein test with a result of 1.5 (range of 0.5 to 5.5), putting me at the low end of the scale of the risk factors for heart disease. Approximately seven years ago, I underwent a heart scan, which is a test that measures calcification in the three main arteries of the heart. Calcification is the early formation of plaque in the arteries. The score can be anywhere from zero to the thousands, depending on the level of calcification. My score was zero, and the report stated that there was no evidence of coronary artery calcification, which suggests a very low likelihood of obstructive coronary artery disease. I have yet to have any doctor capable of explaining how I have experienced almost thirty years of extremely high cholesterol levels and yet have not suffered any damage or plaque buildup in my arteries. One hypothesis is that estrogen prevents the plaque from sticking to the walls of the coronary arteries and instead allows the plaque to easily pass through, preventing any plaque buildup or narrowing of the artery walls.

In my specific example, it can be seen that the importance of the change in today's estrogen recommendations is critical. I personally could suffer major and irreversible health consequences as a result of changing, in any form, my present estrogen medication. All of the previous studies were performed on *older* women, which means that many of the subject's health had already started deteriorating, so there is no evidence of the benefits that estrogen creates in *younger* women. In my specific case, my use of estrogen started early in my life before any deterioration of my health began. Because my hormone levels have remained the same as they were when I was thirty-one, could this be a good example of what has been described as "estrogen protecting women against cardiovascular disease during the childbearing years"?

There is an interesting website listed on the Internet by the National Heart, Lung, and Blood Institute (www.nhlbi.nih.gov/health/women/pht_facts.htm) that describes postmenopausal use of estrogen by stating that "a woman's risk of developing heart disease begins to rise around menopause. After menopause, women's rate of bone loss increases." Further along, it states, "Through the years, studies were finding evidence that estrogen might help with some of these menopausal risks — especially heart disease and osteoporosis." Several paragraphs later, it states, "Many scientists believed these increased health risks were linked to the postmenopausal drop in estrogen produced by the ovaries and that replacing estrogen would help protect against the diseases." Consider the idea that perhaps estrogen should be started *before* any disease starts or health deterioration begins. Maybe that is the area missed concerning the benefits of estrogen. Perhaps estrogen is given too late because disease has already formed. There is no way of knowing because studies have not been performed on young and healthy subjects. In my specific case, estrogen therapy was started *before* any deterioration of my health or disease began, including any narrowing of my coronary arteries.

The American Society for Reproductive Medicine printed an article in Vol. 81, No.6, June 2004, that states, in part:

> Early initiation of estrogen replacement has been shown to inhibit atherosclerosis and the response to vascular injury in a series of animal models. This is not surprising in light of the presence of both estrogen receptors and estrogen synthetase in human coronary vessels. However, recent studies suggest that this benefit is lost if initiation of estrogen replacement is delayed until years after the menopause. This may reflect estrogen's ability to prevent lesion formation but not to prevent

progression of already-established lesions. Therefore, it should not be surprising that salutary effects of estrogen on cardiovascular disease may require early administration and a long observation period before the better-maintained cardiovascular health of the treated women becomes apparent. These observations suggest that the appropriate study group for post-menopausal cardioprotection is newly menopausal women who receive estrogen for some years, as was the case in the observational studies.

2. Digestive Health. I just had a colonoscopy, and the doctor was surprised because my test was absolutely clean. The doctor said people in my age group usually have the beginning symptoms of diverticulitis or polyps. I had neither.

3. Bone Density. I recently had a bone density test, and the results were above average for my age. The actual result was reported as "bone density is up to 10 percent below young normal." It also stated that, "Fracture risk is low." I had never suffered a broken bone in my life until early 2009, when the side of my foot was forcefully slammed into a pointed base of a column after skidding across a slippery surface. Trust me — that incident would have broken the bones of Sampson or Hercules!

4. Breast Cancer. I get mammograms regularly every year. They have always been clear, but I still worry, as my paternal grandmother contracted breast cancer at age sixty-six which was considered "old age onset."

5. Blood Pressure. My blood pressure, on average, is approximately 108/72. During my recent colonoscopy, my blood pressure, which was being monitored regularly throughout the procedure, had readings of 110/58.

6. General Health. I am still enjoying life to the fullest. I feel no different today from the way I felt when I was in my thirties. My energy level is as high as it has been throughout my life, and I have experienced no signs or symptoms of needing to slow down or to change my daily routine. I have enjoyed a very youthful attitude and mindset for my entire life. My face and body have not sustained any major amount of wrinkles. My hair shows no signs of thinning, and in fact, is thicker today than it was five years ago. My eyes still have moisture, which enables me to continue to wear my contact lenses, as I have for almost forty years. My womanly shape has remained the same. My husband and I enjoy our sexual relationship in the same manner that we have for almost forty-three years. Basically, my body has not changed in any area.

I have experienced a lifetime of excellent health. I am sure that my own individual medical experiences will be questioned and challenged; however, my existence validates my claims. Any detrimental health changes that I may sustain in the future can only be considered "old age onset" because I am now sixty-two years old. My experience of a life lived without menopause can be, and should be, a new starting point for the medical community to consider. There is merit in developing a new direction in the prevention of menopause as well as the research of long-term use of estrogen in relation to improved health benefits for women.

Sexual Activity in Postmenopausal Women

What's Sex Got to Do with It?

Another recent issue that has surfaced concerning postmenopausal women is their sexual desire or lack thereof. The medical and pharmaceutical industries are certainly not clear on, and may be oblivious to, the issue of women having their womanhood greatly diminished as a result of menopause and post-menopause syndrome. Both occurrences reduce, if not completely stop, womanly desires and sexual feelings. If I had to experience just one day of achy joints, insomnia, dry eyes and thinning hair, sex would be the last thing on my mind! There needs to be a balancing of the sexual appetites and abilities of both women and men through and past middle age. Amazingly, pharmaceutical companies are scurrying around in an attempt to bridge the gap of difficulty women are having with sexual interest and desire by creating a drug to better enhance their "sexuality." If a woman does not have the estrogen or body fluids necessary in her body to better enhance the sensation, the chance of any drug being able to duplicate such a process could be questionable.

One medical reason women could be disinterested in sexual activities in their later years could be atrophy. Atrophy is a result of menopause. Atrophy occurs when estrogen loss causes tissues of the vulva and the lining of vagina to become thin, dry, and less elastic. Vaginal secretions also diminish, which affects the lubrication process. The loss of estrogen results in a decrease in vaginal fluid, which increases the vaginal pH, which in turn changes a healthy, acidic environment to an alkaline environment, thereby increasing the possibility of vaginal infections. So, if this is what takes place, how are women going to eagerly and enthusiastically have or respond favorably to sexual desires? Vaginal cream is the present proposed remedy. I can remember many years ago reference being made to old women as dried up prunes, and I never understood the reason for using that metaphor. Now that I understand the full gamut of the menopause process, I understand the comparison.

Millions of Baby Boomers, who had discovered sexual freedom with the advantage of the birth control pill and women's liberation during the wild sixties, are not about to dry up like old prunes. Their open attitude is what caused the sexual revolution in the first place. Do you think Baby Boomers are going to take this lying down? Only if she can be on top!

As a matter of fact, The Nassau Guardian reported in August '09 that according to relationship therapist and certified clinical sex therapist, Margaret Bain, a quality sex life for women can be enjoyed later in life with Replacement Hormone Therapy to ensure that the estrogen and testosterone hormone that they — and men — need for sexual desire lasts as long as possible.

With some of the Baby Boomers now becoming respected scientists and sex therapists, we have a good chance at change. Fear is our biggest deterrent. I say, "Bring on the hormones!"

The Comparison: Our Partners vs. Us

Men do not experience the same type of aging process as women. Their manhood remains intact during their lifetime. Even though their sexual capabilities may decline, their body chemistries do not change. Women, on the other hand, undergo a physical change, and their femininity or womanhood decreases as they age. Women lose their actual body fluids and sexual sensations as they age because of the decrease in their estrogen levels.

The pharmaceutical industry seems to be very concerned about men's sexuality in their later years and has introduced three prescription drugs that help to enhance and maintain male sexual performance.

Oddly enough, women's ability to maintain or improve their sexual performance in their later years has not changed at all. The medical industry forgot one very important factor: Women of that age group are not the same as their counterparts. A good example of this specific situation is that you could take a sixty-year-old man and have plastic surgery performed on his face and dye his hair back to its original color and he would resemble the same person he was in his youth inside and outside, except for his energy and strength levels. If you repeated those same procedures on a sixty-year-old woman, the outside would *appear* to be as it was in her youth, but the chemistry on the inside of the woman would have undergone a major drying-out effect long ago, taking her ability to perform and to enjoy her sexuality—the woman's very womanhood and femininity.

A Man Needs to Know!

Men should be just as interested as women in the menopause process, if not more so, because of its actual effects on them. Many marriages encounter serious trouble during the aging process because men have an interest and desire to continue their sexual activity. The problem is often on the other side of the fence as a woman's desire and interest decreases significantly as she goes through the menopause and aging processes. The pharmaceutical and medical industry's remedy for such a dilemma is to create drugs to aid in keeping men sexually active. The real truth of the matter is that they ignored, or did not care equally, about the concerns of women or about preserving a workable and pleasurable marriage environment as a whole.

Women have a great deal of work to do during their lifetimes. They are the nesters and gatherers, they are the keepers, and they are responsible for trying to keep every part of a family going, on time, and in place for a lifetime. After spending approximately twenty years or more keeping the nest warm and functioning, women wake up one day and discover their bodies are stretched from childbirth, that they possibly have increased their weight over the years, that their breasts have lost their youthful shape and that their vaginas are drying out. That being an average and general description of women in their fifties, what positive element from that description is there to entice women to be interested in sexual activity? When a woman looks into the mirror at that age, the image reflected is usually not one to feel good about, let alone one that initiates a sexual sensation or desire. Ask any man and he, generally speaking, will say he would love to have his wife remain physically and mentally youthful, full of energy, and still desirous of him in the same manner as she was at the beginning of their relationship.

<u>Opposite Sides of the Fence</u>

Men, amazingly enough, do not seem to have a similar negative attitude as they age. Their bodies do not undergo the extreme deterioration or major chemistry changes that women's bodies experience. This fact could explain, in part, why the two groups are on opposite sides of the sexual desire fence and the gap continues to widen. When one considers the fact that men can be given pills to better enhance their sexual desires and activities but women are given vaginal cream, one must wonder whether the medical community really thinks that is the answer. Do medical researchers truly believe that this solution will correct the problem of sexuality in aging couples, or are they simply catering to one sex or dealing with one half of the problem?

These enormous differences put men and women into two very different aging groups in the late middle-aged years. The saddest element concerning the deterioration of women's health during their aging years is that *nothing* has ever been done to prevent or improve any one of those important areas.

Feminine Forever
by Dr. Robert A. Wilson

Probably the most controversial book concerning menopause and estrogen, and one in which almost every article and book about estrogen has referenced, is the book *Feminine Forever1*, written in 1966 by Robert A. Wilson, M.D., a New York gynecologist.

Time published an article, which I recently read even though it was written almost ten years ago. The article, The Estrogen Dilemma: America's No. 1 Drug is an Elixir of Youth, but Women Must Decide if it's Worth the Risk of Cancer (June 1995), was my first introduction to Dr. Robert A. Wilson and his many medical theories and opinions concerning estrogen use as described in his book. Dr. Wilson believed that menopause was completely preventable and curable. Further, he believed menopause was "far from being an act of fate or a state of mind — it is in fact a deficiency disease. By way of a rough analogy, you might think of menopause as a condition similar to diabetes." Dr. Wilson believed women should be given hormones throughout their lives in order to gain maximum benefits.

My life basically confirms Dr. Wilson's medical theories and opinions concerning estrogen, its ability to prevent menopause, and its positive benefits to women's health, as stated in his book. My estrogen level has never decreased during my life, and my story confirms each and every one of Dr. Wilson's medical theories relative to supplementing estrogen throughout a woman's life.

Dr. Wilson's book, which introduced that new concept to women, was considered revolutionary when it first came out in 1966. He believed that if women maintained their estrogen levels throughout their lives, they would not suffer menopause or any of its damaging health-related consequences. Further, Dr. Wilson described women who were successful in preventing menopause as women who were fifty but looked like they were thirty, or women of sixty who looked and acted like they were forty, as my case demonstrates.

As a result of Dr. Wilson's clinical cases, he believed it was apparent that menopause was a chemical imbalance similar to the one present in diabetes. Diabetics are given insulin to restore their sugar levels, and estrogen accomplishes the same goal by restoring a woman's estrogen levels. Dr. Wilson believed that with preventative treatment, women could remain feminine, both physically and emotionally, for as long as they lived. Further, he believed the outward appearance of women who maintained their estrogen levels could easily be recognized by their smooth facial skin, muscle tone, and energy levels.

Dr. Wilson believed menopause was curable and that with the prevention of it, all the bodily changes that are normally experienced by women could be reversed, with the exception of fertility. However, in order to prevent menopause, a woman must receive treatment *before* the onset of menopause.

According to Dr. Wilson, women should have the option of remaining feminine forever and selecting that option would increase the happiness of millions of families by maintaining enrichment and harmony in women's marriages. His opinion was that menopause often ruins a woman's character along with her health. He believed menopause affected a woman's complete environment as well as other people within her environment.

An interesting concept of Dr. Wilson's was his view that menopause should be recognized as a major medical problem in society and that the treatment and cure of menopause was a social and moral obligation. From his perspective, menopause should be eliminated so that women could have an enduring feminine role throughout their lives. As an example, he mentioned our cultural climate puts a premium on femininity. The entertainment community—theater, movies, television, etc.—all focus on women's sexuality.

Another interesting area that Dr. Wilson mentioned was how little time doctors undergoing medical training spend studying the subject of menopause. In his book, he reported that no more than thirty minutes of lecture was devoted to the topic of menopause during a doctor's entire medical education.

Dr. Wilson's book shocked everyone because he used the word *castration* to define the actual menopause process. The reason that he chose that specific word was because he believed it was the proper term for a syndrome that deprived a person of sexual functions. He further elaborated by explaining that it makes no difference whether castration is achieved by surgical removal of the genital organs or whether the ovaries die as a result of menopause; the result is the same. In his book, Dr. Wilson also ensured women of "escaping the horror of this living decay" in reference to the prevention of menopause. Both of those radial statements made by Dr. Wilson are still quoted today.

As a way of explaining his new use of the term, Dr. Wilson summarized the effects that castration has on a woman's entire body. The symptoms may vary, but include:

- tissues drying out

- weakened muscles

- sagging skin

- brittle and porous bones that fracture easily; this can lead to dowager's hump

He further mentioned that as a result of lost estrogen, menopausal women lose their immunity to coronary disease and experience abnormal blood pressure, increasing their chances of experiencing heart attacks and strokes.

Another important area affected by castration, according to Dr. Wilson, is the entire genital system, which dries out because of the desiccation of tissues. As an example, Dr. Wilson reported that after castration, a woman's breasts shrink and lose their firmness and that the vagina becomes atrophic and that the brittleness of it can cause chronic inflammation resulting in the skin cracking, which could cause infection, in turn making intercourse impossible.

Dr. Wilson also believed menopause was related to age and that as a result of modern medicine lengthening a woman's life span, medicine should also adjust the "rate of aging to fit the longer life." As an example, Dr. Wilson explained the aging process of a healthy man, noting that a man remains male throughout his life and his sexual desires and means of satisfying them do not change. He further explained that even though a man's sex hormones diminish over the years, his sexuality decreases gradually and without any abrupt interruption, unlike the terrible fate of women.

According to Dr. Wilson, "Estrogen therapy doesn't *change* a woman. On the contrary: *it keeps her from changing.* Therapy does not alter the natural hormone balance. Rather it *restores* the total hormone pattern to the normal, pre-menopausal level." I find it very interesting that absolutely *nothing* has changed for women in this area since his book was written more than forty years ago. Extreme medical advancements have taken place in the areas of heart disease, organ transplants, and numerous other areas, yet there has not been *one* medical advancement or improvement made in the area of menopause.

There are many articles and books that favorably reference Dr. Wilson's *Feminine Forever*, and there are many rebuttals of his theories and views. Even though his theories were never studied or confirmed, Dr. Wilson should at least be given credit for his attempt to find a favorable solution to menopause.

The following is a partial list described by Dr. Wilson of the advantages of maintaining estrogen levels throughout a woman's life, and each point is followed by my own personal experience:

♀ It is the hormone of feminine attraction and well-being.

My feminine attraction continues, even after age sixty, along with my excellent general health and well-being.

♀ It keeps a woman sexually attractive and potent.
I can confirm that this has and is continuing to happen to me.

44

♀ It preserves the strength of her bones.
My recent bone density test revealed that I am above average given my age. The report stated, "Bone density is up to 10% below young normal." It further stated, "Fracture risk is low."

♀ It preserves the glow of her skin and hair.
My skin has been smooth and flawless and has maintained a youthful appearance for thirty years. My hair still has a shine and fullness to it.

♀ It prevents heart disease, high blood pressure, strokes and diabetes from developing.
My cardiologist has advised me that even though I have had high cholesterol for more than thirty years, the estrogen has protected my heart. I have no cardiovascular disease. My blood pressure generally is 108/72. My mother, her brother, and their mother had type II diabetes. I do not have any symptoms of diabetes.

♀ It prevents urinary bladder disease.
I have never had urinary bladder disease.

♀ It prevents the kidneys from losing salt in the urine, which is an important function in the regulation of tissue fluids throughout the body.
I have had no kidney issues.

♀ It motivates women in the areas of work, study and ambition and acts as a natural energizer for their mind and body.
I have had high energy all of my life and continue to have high energy even at age sixty-two.

♀ It gives women self-confidence and the ability to be effective in their problem-solving tasks.
I have always been the resourceful person in our family, and I enjoy the challenge of trying to solve problems.

♀ It helps women to resist both mental and physical fatigue while helping them to maintain emotional self-control.

> *I have never experienced mental or physical fatigue. My life can be described as always being a cup half full rather then half empty.*

♀ It keeps women's emotional reactions in proportion to an occasion without over reacting.
   My life has been lived in an environment of calmness.

Dr. Wilson believed the following to be additional advantages of estrogen use:

♀ Women who maintain their ability to stay estrogen rich throughout their lives remain cancer poor.

♀ Women's breasts remain firm.

♀ Women's vaginas maintain their strength, durability and elasticity.

♀ Women's gums remain healthy.

♀ Women's eyes resist infection.

♀ Women's joints maintain their flexibility.

Due to the fact that my mother underwent a hysterectomy when she was young and I had a similar experience, the topic of menopause was never discussed. Medically speaking, we were both considered surgical menopause patients, which means that our bodies were forced into menopause as a result of the surgery. My mother had her hysterectomy in 1949 and was not given estrogen even though it had been available for seven years. She did experience the typical aging process. My mother contracted pancreatic cancer when she was sixty-eight years old. Ironically, her system had been without estrogen for forty-four years when she contracted the disease, and there has never been any other case of cancer in her family. One of Dr. Wilson's theories was that "women who stay estrogen-rich throughout their lives will remain happily cancer-poor." Is there any correlation? Currently there is no way to know because studies and research have not been conducted among women who have lived any length of their lives, or even the majority of their lives, without estrogen. As an example, if a woman has completed the menopause process by age forty-five (early menopause) and her system is without estrogen for twenty years, will she increase her risk of getting cancer by the time she reaches sixty-five?

According to Dr. Wilson, estrogen affects every cell of the female body and the resulting mental changes totally alter a woman's position relative to her family and herself.

As a summary of Dr. Wilson's medical theories, the following are some of his arguments relative to estrogen use.

1. Menopause is not necessary.

2. Treatment to prevent menopause should begin in a woman's middle thirties, before the onset of menopause.

3. Estrogen acts as a cancer preventive.

4. Menopausal symptoms, including heart trouble, hardening of the arteries, weakening of the bones and muscles, atrophy of the breasts and sexual organs, pains in the joints, impaired vision, and wrinkles of the skin can be avoided by maintaining estrogen.

5. Mental depression can be avoided.

6. Sexual activity and enjoyment can be achieved past middle age.

7. Both youthful appearance and vigorous energy levels are retained.

Dr. Wilson's book, *Feminine Forever,* is still referenced in many articles and books today. His revolutionary concept of eliminating menopause as well as his reference to menopausal women as "castrates" is still considered radical thinking even today, forty-one years after he wrote his book.

However, as radical and difficult as it may be to believe, I am the product of the continued and stable estrogen levels that Dr. Wilson described in his book. I have the youthful appearance that he described could be retained; the outstanding general health; and specifically, the protection of the heart as he described, along with all of the other benefits. More importantly, I have escaped the menopause process as he said could be done—by maintaining my estrogen level throughout my life. My health and medical experiences are parallel to Dr. Wilson's theories regarding every medical issue he listed as areas of concern— heart disease, bone density, wrinkled skin, thinning hair, sagging breasts, and energy levels, just to name a few.

My particular medical situation, while paralleling Dr. Wilson's theories, should not be taken as medical advice in any form. Women have different medical circumstances and only their doctors can give them medical advice relative to their specific requirements.

It must be understood that the estrogen environment, coupled with women's own medical circumstances, are very different and complicated, and each case must be treated individually. That is exactly the point the government has missed relative to the WHI study and the result that followed in assuming that all estrogen users had the same medical situation.

Dr. Wilson outlined his medical theories, statistics, and opinions in his book. However, I am the product of his theories based upon long-term estrogen use, and more importantly, I am the product of a thirty-year study that should obviously have been, but was never funded.

I am not supporting, confirming, or denying any theories or medical statements. I am only bringing about an awareness of a completely different aspect of the complicated estrogen environment for women who may not have all the information. My lifetime of good medical health after taking estrogen alone for almost thirty years should raise many questions about many theories. Hopefully, the exposure of my specific medical situation will create questions and apply pressure to the medical community so they must provide once and for all, to all women of all ages and medical situations, true and accurate medical information concerning hormone replacement therapy.

Shedding Light on the Difference

This book has no objective in referencing Dr. Wilson's book *Feminine Forever* other than comparing my life experiences to his medical theories concerning two major issues: (1) estrogen can be used throughout a woman's life and (2) menopause is preventable. I probably would have been extremely puzzled and disturbed to find out how different I was if I had not read Dr. Wilson's book, which explains the reasons for many events that have occurred in my lifetime. Further, I find it extremely unusual that I mirror Dr. Wilson's medical opinions point for point. Undoubtedly, my situation will be an issue of controversy, but my health and statistics during the past thirty years verify the events.

Since there is no data available on long-term estrogen use, I have created a hyperlink on my website (dwalters@menopausefree.org) requesting women to furnish their experience of long-term estrogen use. I believe the collective data will bring forth interesting and necessary observational data, and this may well be the first database of its kind.

Women's Health Initiative (WHI)

Confusion and Fear

The result of the WHI 2002 study, unfortunately, has created confusion and fear for women using any form of estrogen. Several years ago, the WHI published a twenty-five-page fact sheet which was available on their website (www.whi.org). An interesting sentence on their website stated: "Choosing whether or not to use postmenopausal hormone therapy can be one of the most important health decisions women face as they age. As with taking any treatment, the decision involves carefully weighing the risks and benefits involved." Their website also stated: "Being informed is one of the best ways you can protect your health." This statement is good advice. However, the truth and awful irony of the matter is that based upon the information they furnished to the public, women were not properly or accurately informed to enable them to make the decisions necessary to protect their health. The WHI failed in their attempt to provide accurate information to women through their faulty analysis and data from their very costly ($735 million) study.

Nancy Hicks of the Lincoln Journal Star reported that a national expert in the field of reproductive endocrinology and professor of obstetrics and gynecology, Dr. Leon Speroff said, "Slowly but surely, an accurate assessment of the WHI data has emerged."

"A massive analysis of more than twelve hundred women and six mammography screening centers, published in '08, indicated that women on estrogen-progesterone therapy for five years or more had *reduced* the risk of dying from breast cancer compared with women who had never been on hormone therapy," he said at a conference at the Bryan LGH Medical Center's Institute for Women and Children's health.

My heart is broken to think that millions of women are still reacting to the original '02 WHI announcement.

Comparison is Vital

My paternal grandmother contracted breast cancer when she was sixty-six years old. I was very scared that I, too, would contract the disease. In an attempt to assess my risk of contracting breast cancer based on hereditary factors, I spoke with a doctor who specialized in breast cancer research, and he advised me that her disease was considered "old age onset" cancer because of the age factor and could not be viewed as a hereditary factor. The doctor further stated that once a person nears the age of sixty, most ailments and diseases are then considered "old age onset" based simply on the age factor. Because of the age group (which had an average age of sixty-three) of the subjects used in the WHI study, I wonder if the results of those studies produced true results. How does anyone know if their risks were increased simply based on the fact that they were in the older age group? How can any results be considered accurate unless the same study has been performed on a younger age group of women and the two groups produce two identical (or at the very least similar) results, thus confirming the evidence? I would like to see *one* study in which women participants are middle-aged or younger. This may or may not make a difference in the outcome of the studies, but until the studies take into consideration *every* age group, all studies and results should remain subject to question and should be considered unconfirmed as fact. The natural history of breast cancer must be remembered when hearing study results — it takes approximately seven years for a single cancer cell to progress large enough to show on a mammogram and then another three years before it is large enough to felt on a physician exam.

Placed in Harm's Way

A very scary notion is that if the results of the recent WHI study indicating increased risk of breast cancer were, by any chance, incorrect because of the age group of the women participants (average age of sixty-three), then many women who have stopped taking estrogen because of the findings might actually be doing more harm than good to their health. The International Menopause Society (IMS), in their Position Paper stated, "The Executive Committee of the IMS supports the immediate release of the full database from the estrogen + progestin arm of the WHI and the MWS database for independent review." Many scientists wanted the data to be released so that they could analyze the information themselves, taking into account various factors, to see if the same results would be produced. Clearly, doubt was cast on the results, as announced, by the WHI researchers. How are women ever going to feel confident that the medical advice that they are receiving concerning estrogen is true and accurate without full and complete studies, let alone without full and complete disclosure to these facts? The end result of this wild estrogen disorder is that no one knows what action is safe and correct, and sadly, the result of this situation is that women have now been placed in harm's way because of that study.

In trying to understand the reasoning behind why that particular age group (sixty-three to seventy) of women was selected for the test, the following was the mission statement of WHI which was on their website several years ago:

♀ To address the most common causes of death, disability and impaired quality of life in postmenopausal women. The WHI will address cardiovascular disease, cancer, and osteoporosis. The WHI is a fifteen-year, multi-million dollar endeavor and one of the largest U.S. prevention studies of its kind. The three major components of the WHI are:

♀ A randomized controlled clinical trial of promising but unproven approaches to prevention;

♀ An observational study to identify predictors of disease;

♀ A study of community approaches to developing healthful behaviors.

Their mission statement clearly specifies that the WHI is concerned with women of postmenopausal age, which is approximately fifty years old. My disappointment surfaced when I realized that their concern for women's health issues was focused upon women in their later years and was not necessarily associated with the menopause process itself.

On a separate website, the WHI further stated, "The overall goal of WHI is to reduce coronary heart disease, breast and colorectal cancer, and osteoporotic-fracturers among postmenopausal women via prevention strategies and risk factor identification." They listed the following areas of concern to be:

Osteoporosis

♀ One-sixth of all women will have a hip fracture during their lifetime.

♀ Osteoporotic fractures contribute to increased disability and lessen the quality of life in older women.

♀ Hip fractures are more common than the combined risk of breast cancer, uterine cancer, and cervical cancer.

♀ Fractures occur more frequently in women than men (three to four times more frequently) in those over fifty years of age.

♀ There is limited trial data for women on the effect of calcium and Vitamin D on fracture risk.

Heart Disease in Women

♀ Heart disease is the leading cause of death in postmenopausal women.

♀ Over 240,000 women die of heart attacks each year.

♀ Thirty-three percent of all deaths among U.S. women are due to heart disease.

♀ Approximately one-half of all coronary deaths occur in women.

♀ Long-term clinical trials on hormone replacement therapy and the risk of coronary heart disease among women are lacking.

Breast Cancer

♀ Breast cancer is the second leading cause of cancer deaths in U.S. women.

♀ Over 46,000 women die of breast cancer annually.

♀ Approximately 183,000 new cases of breast cancer are discovered each year.

♀ There is inconclusive data on the effect of dietary fat intake on breast cancer.

♀ There is inconsistent data on the effect of hormones on breast cancer risk.

Colon Cancer

♀ Colon cancer is the third leading cause of cancer deaths in U.S. women.

♀ Over 28,000 women die of colorectal cancer each year.

♀ Approximately 51,000 women per year are diagnosed with colon cancer; 16,500 new cases of rectal cancer are discovered in women each year.

♀ Studies suggest increased calcium and Vitamin D intake may decrease the risk of colorectal cancer."

The WHI states, "*Scientific knowledge about prevention and treatment of diseases common in or unique to women is insufficient. Successful* prevention strategies will have major public health implications." These are the major concerns of the WHI. Again, menopause really is not individually listed in any of their programs as being considered for treatment or research.

Estrogen Plus Progestin

The WHI performed research on two estrogen drugs. One study involved the use of estrogen plus progestin, a combination used by women who have not had a hysterectomy. The second study involved the use of estrogen alone, which is used by women who have had a hysterectomy.

The following is a report of the conclusions of the WHI study. Compared with a placebo, after about five years of use, estrogen plus progestin resulted in alleged increased risks. However, Dr. Crandall and others have re-evaluated the data and evaluated the actual risks. These re-evaluated risks are shown in a separate column on the right.

Increased risks	Actual risks
• 26% increase in breast cancer	**No increased risk**
• 41% increase in strokes	**No increased risk**
• 29% increase in heart attacks	**No increased risk**
• Doubled rates of blood clots in legs and lungs	**Increased risk**

Increased benefits

- 37% less colorectal cancer
- 34% fewer hip fractures

Questions to Think About — Answers to Obtain

I know there are many questions that remain unanswered concerning estrogen. The issues raised by this book will probably complicate matters even more. However, questions concerning estrogen and menopause are never asked in *advance* of the onset of menopause by the younger age group of women who would benefit the most by preventative HRT. We are taught to practice, and our medical delivery system is now focused on, preventative medicine because the end results are more advantageous to our health. Strange, but true, menopause and hormone therapy are two medical areas in which practicing preventive medicine does not apply. The research, results, and recommendations concerning menopause and estrogen have been conducted during and apply to the period of time *after* this major change or detrimental medical event has occurred. Perhaps now would be a good time to redirect the attention and studies in the area of practicing preventative measures concerning menopause and estrogen therapy.

The following is a list of general questions concerning menopause:

1. Is menopause preventable or curable?

2. Have any improvements been made to ease the menopause process?

3. Is menopause a chemistry deficiency within the body that can be corrected?

4. Should estrogen be given as a supplement when the natural levels begin to decrease?

5. As a result of menopause, does a woman's state of health (i) stay the same, (ii) improve, or (iii) deteriorate?

6. What would a woman's state of health be after her body has been without estrogen long-term (ten to fifteen years) and even longer (twenty-five years) and does it matter?

7. What is the risk, if any, of a woman contracting cancer as a result of her body being without estrogen for a long period of time?

8. Regarding clinical studies and research:

   a. What is the average age of participants?

   b. Why haven't studies been performed on the younger population?

   c. Why hasn't research been recorded on women who have had hysterectomies and who have been taking estrogen for twenty years or longer?

9. Why haven't there been any studies and research in the actual area of *prevention* of menopause?

10. If Viagra is the answer for sexual dysfunction for the male population, what is the answer for the sexual dysfunction of the female?

11. As a result of the pandemonium and mass confusion in the now dangerous environment concerning the use of estrogen, should an independent organization be created (such as a Women's Bureau of Medical Affairs) to help in the following areas:

    a. Address the important issues of women's health needs.

    b. Provide current information concerning women's health issues.

    c. Stabilize and regulate the mismanaged estrogen environment.

    d. Attempt to clarify estrogen controversies.

e. Seek funding for trials and research.

f. Centralize and provide current information and news releases for the public.

Who Has the Answer?

<u>Turning Point</u>

I recently had my annual physical with my doctor, who is a well-respected female general internist in the suburbs of Washington, D.C. After reviewing all of the results of my tests (complete blood count, EKG, mammogram, colonoscopy, and bone density test), all of which were perfect, my doctor raised the issue of hormone replacement therapy. She mentioned the fact that I had been taking estrogen for almost thirty years, and she wanted me to consider stopping the use of it. When I was evasive concerning the topic, she further mentioned, as an alternative, the possibility of reducing the dosage of estrogen that I had been taking all these years. I asked her what that might do for my health, and she stated that it could, among other things, produce hot flashes. She also said that because I was still sexually active, I could possibly experience symptoms of vaginal dryness. I was surprised by her recommendation as I have never experienced one symptom of menopause, and my life has not changed in any manner during the past thirty years. However, she thought it would be advantageous for me to stop taking estrogen and did not elaborate on any additional specific details. What my doctor didn't know during this extensive physical exam was that I had gained valuable knowledge of the many benefits of taking estrogen for the long-term.

At the conclusion of the consultation, I advised my doctor that I would continue taking Premarin and would not consider reducing the dosage. I did find it strange, however, that I was making a medical decision concerning my health instead of feeling confident about my doctor's medical opinion concerning this issue. Since that time, many women have told me that they have regretted not being more informed concerning the important estrogen issues, and as a result, their health has diminished.

I left my doctor's office very confused and wondered why she would want to change my state of excellent health to one of a declining health. What medical advantage would there be to having hot flashes or any other menopausal symptoms as I entered my sixties? I thought about the situation in a more important manner: Would I be healthier if I stopped the use of estrogen or if I continued the use of estrogen? How frightening to me to know that although I had walked into my doctor's office having **experienced excellent health for sixty-two years**, that fact could have changed drastically because of the most current medical recommendations concerning hormone replacement therapy. Due to inaccurate and flawed information, I faced the possibility of suffering irreversible medical consequences.

The possibility of what could have happened to me clearly documents the importance of the estrogen environment as a whole rather than just the concerns of the postmenopausal group of women who are always referenced. Reiterating, the medical cases concerning women who have been taking estrogen alone for longer than twenty years is completely different from those of the postmenopausal women who take hormones for the relief of menopause symptoms for approximately five years or less.

♀ This group of women has been taking estrogen alone long-term as a result of undergoing hysterectomies (including ovaries) prior to the onset of menopause.

♀ These women are referred to as "surgical menopause patients"; the surgery immediately induces menopause, regardless of age.

♀ They are then given estrogen alone to stop the process from continuing, and they remain on hormones for an indefinite period of time.

♀ There is no recommended length of treatment, no dosage amount, and no regulations for those women who have remained, and continue to remain, on estrogen alone long-term.

♀ The FDA's current recommendation for taking estrogen at the lowest dosage for the shortest period of time DOES NOT apply to this group and could result in medical harm.

<u>Why Change?</u>

This particular group of women is isolated by what has happened to them, and yet there is the chance that any one of them could be given the wrong medical information based upon today's current recommendations for using estrogen. How can any medical professional who has previously advised and prescribed estrogen alone to women for more than twenty years, with successful results, suddenly change his or her position? What medical changes would occur to these women who have been successfully taking estrogen alone long-term? Would their state of health remain the same, improve, or deteriorate? Would the change place them into an immediate state of irreversible menopause? What side effects would surface as a result of stopping the use of hormones after such a lengthy period of time?

The FDA, the National Institutes of Health (NIH) and the WHI could be considered irresponsible in making a general statement of recommendations concerning the dosage and length of treatment for *all* women who are presently taking estrogen. Without studying, or at least giving consideration to the extremely different set of circumstances of all the women taking estrogen, their conclusions are encompassed by controversy. Equally important they are making the general statement of recommendations *without knowing in advance* what the results and effects of changing the dosage and length of treatment of hormones, if any, would be. Would the changes in both the dosage and length of treatment (from twenty or more years to less than five years) result in serious and irreversible medical harm? This new change of recommended dosage and length of treatment for using estrogen is a direct result of the study performed by the WHI; however, that study did not include data regarding women who had been taking estrogen alone for twenty years or longer. How can the new recommendations be *safely and correctly* applied to this group of women without that knowledge? What does the research data state regarding this specific group of women? Who is responsible for making this medical decision in the event that the changes that take place are irreversibly detrimental to the health of this group of women?

Linda's Story

Linda, the wife of one of my co-workers, had a hysterectomy about fifteen years ago. She had been taking estrogen alone. Because of the recent WHI study results, doctors recommended that she stop her usage of estrogen. Using her specific situation as an example, who can tell her what harm or good, if any, she will experience as a result of stopping her long-term use of estrogen alone? More importantly, the following questions surface: What is medically happening to her body now that she has not taken estrogen for more than two years? Is it creating any significant changes to her body to the point where she will *not* be able to resume taking estrogen? How much time can lapse before it is considered too late to resume taking estrogen in the event that ceasing usage was the wrong decision? These are just a few of the many important questions relative to women taking estrogen alone, but there are no answers to give the women who have been, and presently continue, taking estrogen alone long-term. Who can these women, having taken estrogen alone long-term, turn to in order to get the answers needed concerning their specific cases. Who can help them make the best informed medical decisions to protect their health? How can these women make safe and informed decisions concerning their health when there has not been any research conducted—much less any answers discovered—for this specific group?

Another Example

Another similar situation is that of a woman who was a surgical menopause patient many years ago and is also a long-term user of estrogen alone. She, too, based upon the medical advice of her doctor, stopped taking estrogen alone because of the new recommendations to take the lowest dosage for the shortest period of time. Her health quickly deteriorated in many areas, and as a result she returned to her doctor and *demanded* that she be able to resume taking estrogen alone, which she had been on for more than twenty years. As a result of resuming her original treatment of estrogen alone, she immediately experienced improvements and eventually regained her good general health status.

My recent doctor's visit, as well as the two similar cases of these women, reflects the important, yet unknown, territory concerning the women who have been using estrogen alone long-term. All of these women were advised to stop using estrogen alone after having taken the hormone for a very long time. These examples clearly demonstrate:

1. The medical importance and neglect of the group of women who have been using estrogen alone for the long-term without any controversy. If usage is just now being labeled as harmful, what happens to the millions of women who have been taking it for more than thirty years? Instead, all within one day and one study, women have been given the wrong medical advice?

2. The detrimental medical effect that today's new recommendations concerning estrogen have had regarding long-term estrogen alone cases.

Two HRT Regimens

The two hormone replacement regimens, estrogen alone and estrogen plus progestin, are different and are used for different circumstances. However, the manner in which the WHI study results were announced, categorized, and presented to the general public indicates all women who were taking any form of estrogen were considered to have the same set of medical circumstances. Could such a situation cause irreversible harm to the many women who have been taking estrogen for longer than twenty years?

Important Differences

Noting my specific medical situation is that of a woman whose body has **never started** the menopause process is vitally important. That difference is necessary since most references to trials, studies, results, and recommendations associated with menopause deal with women whose bodies **have started** the menopause process. Moreover, estrogen is generally referenced as being used *in conjunction with* the menopause process in an effort to alleviate the uncomfortable side effects that are sometimes experienced as a result of menopause. Most of the media coverage concerning estrogen is associated with menopause symptoms and women of menopausal age.

The estrogen I have been taking was given to me **before** the menopause process began so my body has **never started** the menopause process. I have never been advised by a doctor to either stop or reduce my dosage until the WHI study results were announced, so I have taken the same amount of estrogen for thirty years, which means I have never had any decline in my estrogen level, as the chart below illustrates. The question is: what medical changes occur to a woman's body during the twenty year period from the age of 30 to 50?

Illustration of Estrogen Levels

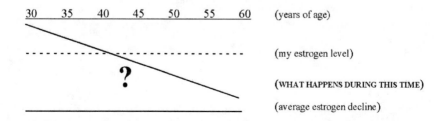

| 30 | 35 | 40 | 45 | 50 | 55 | 60 | (years of age) |

(my estrogen level)

?

(WHAT HAPPENS DURING THIS TIME)

(average estrogen decline)

I believe this is a very important difference, but again, there is no medical evidence, no studies, no data, and no research to clarify or explain what, if any, differences exists between women who started taking estrogen *before* the onset of the menopause process and women who started menopause and used estrogen to alleviate the side effects.

Estrogen has been in the marketplace for sixty-five years. Such a time span should have been sufficient to research hormones in order to know what risks and/or benefits, if any, they create. Without this information, the hormone replacement environment continues to be very dangerous and unsafe for women.

Understanding the WHI Estrogen Plus Progestin Study

Dr. Crandall

In order to better understand the study, we will briefly review the methods used, the statistics, and the pharmacology of the hormones used. The natural history of the diseases will be discussed separately. This study recruited postmenopausal women to be in the largest randomized study on hormone use ever undertaken. Originally, it was thought that it would be double blind (neither patient nor prescriber knows who gets the active hormone). The designers of the study (an epidemiologist and two statisticians) did not realize that most women and their health care providers would know if they were on the active hormone within days or weeks of starting the hormones. This means that it was actually a randomized, partially blind study. The dose used would cause a significant change in most women that would not be present in the placebo group. There were over eight thousand women in each group in the first year, but only about eight hundred remained in the hormone group, and only about five hundred in the placebo group, in the sixth year. The women were incredibly well randomized, with almost exactly the same percentages of women with high blood pressure, diabetes, high cholesterol, history of stroke, heart attack, and blood clots in both groups.

Statistics are difficult to understand, and most people do not read the statistical analyses of an article. The second paragraph of the statistical analyses beginning on page 325 should be read slowly and carefully. Below is the paragraph with commentary in italics.

"Two forms of CIs are presented, nominal and adjusted."
*CIs are confidence intervals. If the CI does not cross 1.0,
then the finding is statistically significant. Statistically
significant does not necessarily mean important or correct.*
"Nominal 95% CIs describe the variability in the
estimates that would arise from a simple trial for a
single outcome. Although traditional, these CIs do not
account for the multiple statistical testing issues (across
time and across outcome categories) that occurred in
this trial, so the probability is greater than .05 that at
least 1 of these CIs will exclude unity under an overall
null hypothesis. The adjusted 95% CIs presented herein
use group sequential methods to correct for multiple
analyses over time."

*This says that according to the WHI statisticians, the adjusted CIs
should be used, not the nominal or unadjusted CIs. The last sentence in
the paragraph seems to disagree.* "This report focuses primarily on results
using the unadjusted statistics and also relies on consistency across
diagnostic categories, supportive data from other studies, and biologic
plausibility for interpretation of the findings." *What does "consistency
across diagnostic categories" mean? Why should it matter if different
diagnostic categories come out the same or different? What do other studies
have to do with this study? "Biologic plausibility" can only mean what the
authors thought would happen.*

When the study was completed and there were only two significant
adjusted CIs, (deep vein blood clots were increased [CI 1.14–3.74] and
other osteoporotic fractures decreased [CI 0.63–0.94]), a decision was
apparently made to use the unadjusted, or nominal, CIs despite the
statisticians' recommendations. There is a perception in the lay public
as well as the scientific community that there being no significant result
indicates a failed study. Far from indicating a failed study, it just means
that nothing bad or good happened during the time the study was
performed. If you understand the pharmacology of the hormones used,
observe the results over time, and understand the natural history of
the diseases being followed, then even if the unadjusted statistics are
used, the outcome is expected with the correct conclusions that were
discussed earlier.

The pharmacology of oral hormones is quite interesting. When taken orally, all medications are absorbed in the stomach or small intestine. The oral hormone then passes through the liver. As hormones, including birth control pills, pass through the liver, they induce the liver to produce:

clotting factors
hypertensive factors
migraine factors
diabetic factors

This is not a reason for most women not to take oral hormones or oral birth control pills. If you have any condition or increased risk that would be made worse or would be brought on by these factors, then another route of delivery that bypasses the liver would be better. Other methods would be skin patches, gels, creams, or lotions. Vaginal rings, gels, creams, and tablets would also bypass the liver.

Premarin was used in this study because it was the most widely prescribed hormone in use when the study was designed. Premarin was one of the first oral estrogens available for women. It was the only choice for years, and millions of women took it or are continuing to take it. There is no reason to stop or change it if a woman is having no problems and has no reason to change to another route of delivery. Most women in this study should not have been prescribed oral hormones. Ninety-five percent had absolute or relative reasons not to take oral hormones.

Groups of Estrogen Users

Donna Walters

With regard to estrogen levels and use, women using estrogen can generally be categorized into one of the following four groups:

1. **_Women without surgical change._** This group is comprised of women who are proceeding through life without any surgical change to their reproductive organs. They will enter the menopause process in a natural state. Because these women still have their uteri, they are candidates for the estrogen plus progestin treatment for the purpose of easing menopausal symptoms; the general length of time of treatment for that purpose is now two to three years. This group of women **will** experience menopause *if they follow the current recommendations.*

2. **_Women without uteri._** This group is comprised of women who have had their uteri removed without their ovaries being removed. This means that their ovaries keep producing estrogen on a normal basis. They too will enter the menopause process in a natural state. Because these women do not have their uteri, they are candidates to use estrogen alone for the purpose of easing menopausal symptoms; the general length of time for treatment for that purpose is now two to three years. This group of women **will** also experience menopause *if they follow the current recommendations.*

3. **_Women taking oral contraceptives._** This group is comprised of women who are taking birth control pills, which contain estrogen. They will continue having a menstrual period, which will eliminate the

menopause process or any symptoms of it as long as they remain on the drug. There are no guidelines or recommendations in place regarding how long this group of women should remain on birth control pills. This group of women **will not** experience menopause as long as they are taking birth control pills.

4. ***Women without uteri and ovaries.*** This group is comprised of women who have had a hysterectomy to remove both their uteri and ovaries. As a result, they are considered "surgical menopause patients" and are given estrogen alone to prevent the onset of the menopause process. This group of women have had a hysterectomy (which can be performed at any age), and as a result, they will remain on estrogen alone for an extended period of time. There are no guidelines or recommendations in place regarding how long this group of women should remain on estrogen alone. Similarly to those who take birth control pills, this group of women also **will not** experience menopause as long as they remain on estrogen.

A spokesperson at the WHI reported there are approximately nineteen million women who are taking estrogen. The spokesperson further advised that the new recommended guidelines concerning estrogen specifically targeted and were directed at women who were taking estrogen plus progestin. The news media was not clear in that regard because the recommendations that were announced concerned estrogen use in general; this caused the medical state of confusion that everyone is experiencing today, which could result in harmful medical consequences.

The following graph shows how all four groups of women are distinctly different and illustrates each group's circumstances in taking the different forms of estrogen. It further shows that women in Group 3 and Group 4 experience no change in their estrogen levels as long as they continue use of the different forms of estrogen, even long-term.

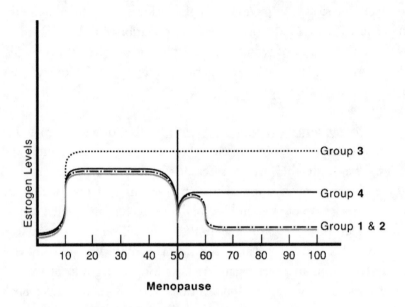

Menopause

--- Group **1**: women without surgical change

─── Group **2**: women without a uterus

······ Group **3**: women taking oral contraceptives

─── Group **4**: women without uterus and ovaries

Estrogen and Its Effect on Other Parts of the Body

Donna Walters

The following articles confirm Dr. Wilson's theories relative to estrogen use and the ways estrogen affects different parts of the body. I can confirm that each one of the following areas describes my specific medical situation.

Estrogen and the Heart

An article on the internet (http://www.holistic-online.com April 19, 2005) about cardiovascular diseases states:

> For reasons unknown, estrogen helps protect women against CVD during the childbearing years.
>
> This is true even when they have the same risk factors as men, including smoking, high blood cholesterol levels, and a family history of heart disease. But the protection disappears when the women go through menopause. After menopause, the incidence of CVD increases, with each passing year posing a greater risk.
>
> Menopause brings changes in the level of fats in a woman's blood. LDL cholesterol appears to increase while HDL decreases in

postmenopausal women as a direct result of estrogen deficiency. Elevated LDL and total cholesterol levels can lead to stroke, heart attack, and death.

Could this be the reason why my arteries have remained open and without plaque buildup despite twenty-five years of high (477) cholesterol levels? Is the result that I have experienced for the past thirty years due to my system maintaining the same levels of estrogen that I had during my childbearing years? Will I experience this benefit as long as I continue to take estrogen? What would happen to my coronary arteries if I stopped taking estrogen alone? If I stopped taking estrogen alone for any length of time, could I recapture the protection if I resumed taking estrogen alone at a later time or would damage have already started and, if so, could it be reversed by taking estrogen alone?

For years women have had to take their seat in the back of the bus when it comes to heart disease.

♀ Nearly two-thirds of deaths from heart attacks in women occur among those who have had no history of chest pain.

♀ Studies show that women who are eligible candidates to receive life-saving, clot-buster drugs are far less likely than men to receive them.

♀ Since 1984, more women than men have died each year from heart disease, and the gap between men and women's survival continues to widen.

♀ Men's plaque distributes in clumps whereas women's distributes more evenly throughout, making it harder for physicians to recognize the presence of heart attacks because "characteristic" patterns of chest pain and EKG changes are less frequently present.

♀ A number of studies indicate that estrogen therapy very likely does reduce heart disease in women under sixty.

Estrogen and the Brain

An article (http://web.sfn.org/content/Publications/BrainBriefings/ estrogen.html) listed on the website of the Society of Neuroscience states that research shows that estrogen boosts a variety of brain abilities, including memory.

> Now studies suggest the hormone also is needed to preserve certain brain functions. Men have about half the amount of estrogen as women — the male hormone testosterone is converted into estrogen in the brain — but their supply never completely diminishes.

New research is leading to:

♀ An understanding of how estrogen interacts with other chemicals to carry out many tasks.

♀ Insight on how memories are made and how dementia is born.

♀ The development of customized estrogen-type drugs that act on the brain.

♀ Researchers are also uncovering the many players that interact with estrogen to help it carry out its actions. For example, researchers have found that a group of neurons, which are often damaged in Alzheimer's disease (AD), have receptors for both estrogen and a neuron-protecting chemical known as a nerve growth factor. This suggests that estrogen interacts with the chemical to protect neurons and possibly prevent AD.

♀ Scientists are also finding evidence that estrogen may regulate other proteins that have been directly linked to AD as well as molecules specifically tied to memory.

♀ Researchers hope to develop ways to cause selected benefits of estrogen in the brain. In addition to mental function, estrogen also may affect mood and brain blood flow. Once the hormone's mechanisms are better understood, scientists plan to develop estrogen-like drugs that target specific brain actions.

I have maintained a youthful mindset and a positive and happy attitude for the past thirty years. Are these characteristics a result of the above-referenced benefits of estrogen in the brain affecting "mood and brain blood flow"? Would my personality traits change if I stopped taking estrogen alone?

Estrogen and the Skin

The American College of Obstetricians and Gynecologists have an article in Vol. 104, No. 4 (Supplement), October 2004, on estrogen associated changes of skin which states:

> Estrogen and Skin Aging. There have been only two randomized, double-blinded, placebo-controlled trials that have examined the effects of estrogen therapy (ET) or hormone therapy (HT) on skin. Both trials suggest that ET increases dermis thickness, whereas HT can increase skin collagen fibers.

An article concerning estrogen and skin (http://www.skinbiology. com/menopause&aging.html) states:

> The drop in estrogen production makes your skin thinner and less elastic, which produces more wrinkling and sagging. Your skin is producing less collagen and elastin, the supportive and elastic proteins in the skin. Again estrogen replacement therapy works to maintain more adequate production of collagen and elastin.

> A 1997 study of 3,875 postmenopausal women concluded that the estrogen helped aging women have a younger looking skin, helped maintain skin's collagen, thickness, elasticity and ability to retain moisture. The study found that the chances of having dry and wrinkled skin were 30 percent less in women who took estrogen replacements in comparison with women who did not. While smoking and sun exposure may

adversely affect skin health, the researchers adjusted for these two factors, and found the benefits of estrogen on skin health were still significant. The study, led by Dr. Laura B. Dunn of the University of California at San Francisco, was published in the Archives of Dermatology (1997; 133:339-342). The researcher commented, "skin wrinkling can negatively affect psychological well-being, sometimes initiating a vicious cycle of diminished self-care leading to deteriorating outcomes."

Commenting on the study, Dr. Fran Kaiser, director of the menopause clinic at St. Louis University School of Medicine in Missouri said, "When estrogen is good for your heart, good for your bones, promotes vaginal lubrication, protects against incontinence and now is good for the skin, how can you knock it? There are so many good reasons to support estrogen use. This is one extra-added bonus."

What woman, in today's youthful society, wants less-than-perfect skin? If you live in Beverly Hills or Dallas or Jersey and want to be equal to the rest of the contemporary Boomer Women, you'll probably be tempted to get your aging, run-away skin in control. The knife is their prairie's home companion. Women fearing rejection are willing to do anything to look younger. What if they knew how good their skin could look if they kept with an estrogen replacement regimen?

One of the most obvious physical differences between me and other women of my age group is my skin and the lack of facial wrinkles. I have experienced extensive sun exposure during my lifetime and still have not suffered any permanent skin damage. Was the thirty years of estrogen use the reason for not sustaining the normal aging changes?

Estrogen and the Hair

An article on the Internet (http://www.skinbiology.com/menopause&aging.html) concerning estrogen and hair states:

> Menopause changes the balance between your body's levels of female hormones and male hormones (androgens) which in turn affects your hair. There is a relative increase in the level of male hormones in your body due to the decrease in estrogen. At times, the fine, light hairs covering your face tend to darken and thicken. Estrogen therapy will reduce this excessive hair growth.
>
> The hair on your scalp begins to thin, as does that hair in the pubic area. Estrogen replacement therapy reduces this hair thinning.

The hair on my scalp has never started to experience the thinning process. Would I experience the normal thinning of hair if I stopped my usage of estrogen? Will my hair maintain its thickness throughout the rest of my life as long as I remain on estrogen alone?

Estrogen and the Eyes

The Doctor's Guide to the Internet (http://www.docguide.com) published an article on June 9, 1997, stating that estrogen may benefit the eyes.

> A study in the June issue of "Ophthalmology" found a reduced incidence of lens opacities, precursors of age-related cataract, in postmenopausal women taking estrogen.

> Although hardening and clouding of the eye's lens occur normally with age, a cataract is characterized by excessive lens opacity. One of the leading causes of blindness in the United States, age-related cataract affects approximately 13 million Americans age 40 and older. Scientists have long suspected that hormones may play a role in the development of age-related cataract because the condition is more common in women than in men.

> Researchers examined the eyes of study participants using fluorophotometry, a technique used to determine the rate of fluid flow in the eye. They found that the group of women taking estrogen had significantly decreased lens opacity relative to the other two groups.

> "These data are suggestive of a beneficial effect of postmenopausal estrogen use on lens transmission in women," the authors concluded, adding, "A protective effect of estrogens on lens transparency could have beneficial effects on qualify of life for older women and would have implications for providing ophthalmic care."

I have not experienced any decrease of eye fluid. In fact, I am still wearing contact lenses with the same prescription that I have worn for the past thirty years. Would my eyes dry out, preventing me from being able to wear contact lenses, if I stopped taking estrogen alone? Would my only option be to resume wearing glasses, which I have not worn since I was fifteen?

Men's Role in Women's Menopause

Men — You Have to Know the Facts

This chapter is about the men's role in the women's menopause process, or the lack of it, as has been the case for a substantial majority of men. It is not about the theory of male menopause, which is another topic and is not covered in this book.

Both disheartening and sad are the many jokes made, primarily by males, about the menopause process. If men were educated, and knew the facts, then perhaps they wouldn't be as inclined to consider the subject as funny and degrading.

Men do not experience chemistry changes within their bodies similar to those in women undergoing menopause. Hence, many of the changes and results that women sustain as a result of menopause are foreign and not understood by men. Many men are probably unfamiliar with the actual process of menopause — what medically takes place; how long the process lasts; and more importantly, the seriousness of the event and the adverse effect it can have on women and any relationship they may be part of at that time. There are many marriages that break up after a lifetime as a result of the extreme changes that take place in a woman's body during the menopausal years. The chance exists that neither the husband nor wife is fully aware of the impact and result that menopause creates for the couple as a unit.

Generally speaking, women do not share their change of life experiences with their significant other. Decisions concerning menopause need to be made in advance of the process, and men are usually not included in the topic of menopause, let alone any part of the decision-making process concerning the matter.

Kissing Femininity Good-bye

Women's sexual sensations are a result of female hormones that develop at puberty and when depleted, the end result is lack of desire and zero interest in sexuality. Hence, I have coined the phrase, "What puberty giveth, menopause taketh away!" Indeed, in many cases, menopause is the death of a woman's femininity. Morever, women often feel that after being married for most of their lives and raising children, the "reward" of menopause is the final blow that extinguishes any spark of interest in sex. In essence, the menopause process ultimately takes women out of the game-of-life. However, as men reach their fifties, they are still very much sexually active. They probably are not fully aware of what has just happened to their significant other and are perplexed as to why their mates find them uninteresting and undesirable in the same sexual manner that was, for the most part, maintained throughout their lives.

Both men and women want to be desired and enjoy the game of anticipation and satisfaction in their relationship. The trouble is, men can continue living in that fashion throughout their lives, and women can only do so for about fifty years. Coupled with that significant problem is the fact that men often don't understand or help women as they undergo the menopause process. The result: two people who share years together and then wake up one day to find that one partner has undergone a significant bodily change while the other partner wonders what in the world has happened.

Lending Men a Helping Hand

If men read this book, I hope the information will help them to understand more fully the changes that take place as women age and approach menopause. Even though menopause only affects the woman directly, and some more severely than others, her entire environment is also affected, including that of her significant other. Many women and men are not fully aware that choices can be made relative to the menopause process and that those choices must be made in a timely manner.

Men, just as women, need to understand and become knowledgeable of the medical process women go through as they age. Men need to understand that women's health issues are complicated, but more importantly, they need to understand that the aging process of women is extremely different from the aging process of men and involves far more than women just "having a bad day." Men need to understand that a woman's body undergoes a major physical and chemical change. Perhaps this book will lend a helping hand to both men and woman in providing them with an awareness of the aging process of women, the options that are available, and — with hope — a better understanding of a man and woman's relationship as it changes through the menopausal years and the many years beyond.

The North American Menopause Society

"The North American Menopause Society (NAMS) is the leading nonprofit organization dedicated to promoting the health and quality of life of women through an understanding of menopause. Its multidisciplinary membership of 2,000 leaders in the field—including clinical and basic science experts from medicine, nursing, sociology, psychology, nutrition, anthropology, epidemiology, pharmacy, and education—allows NAMS to be uniquely qualified to provide information that is both accurate and unbiased, not for or against any point of view." This impressive statement on NAMS' website is very inspiring to a woman in search of answers.

On the same website, NAMS also has a good information sheet pertaining to menopause. Organized in a user-friendly format, five main categories are listed with general questions and responses to the same. The categories are as follows:

1) *Menopause Basics*

2) *Body Changes Around Menopause*

3) *Serious Health Issues at Menopause*

4) *Hormone Therapy Basics*

5) *Achieving Optimal Health*

Their attempt to inform women is admirable. However, my immediate attention went to their list of **eighteen negative health consequences** that could result from experiencing menopause, which are as follows:

Hot flashes	Urine leakage
Sleep pattern changes	Knee aches
Vaginal dryness	Sagging skin
Tiredness	Thinning hair
Headaches	Itching eyes
Memory loss	Tearing eyes
Moodiness	Teeth sensitivity
Depression	Weight gain
Sexual desire decrease	Receding gums

Further to my dismay, was the addition of **four serious health issues** at menopause — **heart disease, diabetes, osteoporosis and cancer.** Yet, under their heading, "Achieving Optimal Health," NAMS states, in part, ***"But, for all women, menopause can mark the beginning of an exciting new time of life."***

I analyzed their data and tried diligently to comprehend why a "stamp of approval" was given for women of menopausal age to sustain such assaults on their well-being. How can a woman's health deteriorate in any of the twenty-two areas (around the age of 51) and those changes then "mark the beginning of an exciting new time of life"? Clearly, NAMS is trying to present menopause in a positive light. However, are they actually advising that the medical consequences that can occur as a result of menopause comprise a healthy and beneficial state for senior women?

In regards to their last category of "Achieving Optimal Health" — the question surfaces as to how could optimal health be accomplished if any, or all, of the eighteen to twenty-two negative health changes have taken place? Twenty-two health changes are major and I personally would rather not put myself into that possible harmful environment as the risks, alone, are frightening. Just when, in our medical environment, was it deemed acceptable for negative health changes to be considered "the beginning of an exciting new time of life"?

Under their section, A Time of New Beginnings, (http://www.menopause.org/expertadvice.aspx, pages 62-63), the opening statement states, "Menopause is a fact of life that affects every woman around the world." However, they failed to mention that millions of women have **not** experienced menopause. These women elected long-term estrogen use in some form, i.e., taking oral contraceptives for twenty, thirty or forty years. Hence, not **every** woman is affected by menopause.

Their second paragraph states, "In today's youth-obsessed society, a woman's perception of menopause can be influenced by many negative stereotypes— in the media, from friends, family, peers and even healthcare professionals." So which is it, a "woman's perception" or the reality of those "twenty-two negative" health risks formulating perceptions?

In their fifth paragraph, they also state, "As women experience the physical, emotional, and social changes of approaching menopause, each woman faces a unique opportunity to identify her own strategies for midlife wellness." Interesting that there was not **one** positive item in their statement. Rather an attitude of trying to have women fix their own menopausal issues was evident. Their suggestion that menopause is "an ideal time to begin or reinforce a health promotion program that will provide benefits through the rest of a woman's life" was clever.

Menopause, with its accompanying health risks, is a very important issue. The suggestion that its arrival ushers in the "beginning of a health promotion program" is an insult to our intelligence. **Prevention** of those health risks is the only answer to menopause and nothing short of that will alleviate or lessen the lifelong damage that can result from menopause!

Sixty-Five Years Later

Impetus for Change — Sixty-five Years and Still Counting

This book is not intended to make women think that they can run to the nearest doctor to seek estrogen and get the same result that I have been fortunate enough to attain during my lifetime. Each woman's situation is going to be different concerning the complicated process of menopause and the related hormones. The purpose of this book is to show that my long-term use of estrogen and my life without menopause are actually good things that produced a positive result, and perhaps the good of it should promote the consideration of taking a new direction in helping women to maintain their womanhood throughout their lives. Women's medical issues are very complicated. Yet, the time is now to realistically address these issues and find resolutions based on women's needs in today's world.

Believing that sixty-five years have passed since estrogen was introduced into the marketplace is difficult and yet the following issues are still controversial and unresolved:

- ♀ Contradiction of hormone studies and their results

- ♀ No resolution or undisputed guidelines and practices concerning hormone therapy protocol and regimen

- ♀ No advancement or change in the menopause process

- ♀ No research or studies aimed at preventing menopause

The hormone replacement therapy dilemma is very complicated and without resolution and is an event that will affect every woman during her lifetime. Yet, we are presently not aware of any doctor, institution, or organization that holds the answer to one very important question:

What is the best and safest medical procedure to follow?
No one has been able to answer that question for the past sixty-five years.

Push Us to the Top!

From the material and information that I have seen, perhaps the issues surrounding menopause are just not important enough for our medical environment to consider them as top-priority. Everyone involved — women, doctors, and researchers — is seemingly satisfied with allowing nature's way to continue without challenge — from inception to the present. Men do not have their sexuality abruptly disappear; however, the medical environment showed interest and concern for men's ability to continue to sexually function in their later years and as a result, quickly created drugs like Viagra. Meanwhile, nothing was introduced into the marketplace to help women in the same regard. A women's femininity and libido gradually deteriorate, and not one new drug has been created to either stop or delay the process. The medical industry's answer is just now surfacing in the form of an attempt to create a drug to increase women's libido levels. A woman's womanhood involves far more than her libido level. If the estimates are true in the latest project concerning libido drugs, the revenue generated from sales of the female libido project — $400 million to $1 billion — should help to get the attention of the pharmaceutical companies and others and prompt them to deal with women's very important health issues. Assuming that these figures are verified, additional research in these areas should be promoted, which in turn, could help to find the answers for all women, including the Forgotten Few.

Now that I have written this book, I have a completely different outlook concerning my physical and mental health. I have an overwhelming sense of appreciation and gratitude concerning my physical being. I cannot truly relate to the experiences of women going through menopause. I hear the words described to me by women and I know and understand the definitions of the adjectives used, but I am unable to relate in a personal way to the physical changes. The closest I have come to a hot flash was a second-hand experience. A co-worker grabbed my hand, put it upon her forehead and said, "This is what a hot flash feels like." I was in total disbelief as the touch of the heat was God-awful. I know that my specific example cannot be followed by all women because I have had a hysterectomy (including the removal of my ovaries). However, there are other women who have similar success stories, so I feel that more attention should be directed to this area to gain valuable information with the hope and expectation of benefiting women throughout their lifetimes.

The medical industry has been accepting and complacent regarding the old-fashioned menopause process rather than rejecting and challenging. The single fact that not one change—not one improvement—has been made since the creation of estrogen sixty-five years ago speaks for itself. Menopause affects, both directly and indirectly, every aspect of a woman's life, be it her own happiness, her marriage, her children and family, or even her work environment. How could something that can affect so many important areas and have a lasting effect on *all* women not be important enough to address, seek positive alternatives to, and change?

One Fact I Know Is True

I cannot dispute or confirm anything involving tests, research, drugs, or opinions. The only fact that I know to be true is that I have spent close to half of my life, almost 30 years, taking an estrogen replacement, specifically Premarin. My lifetime of excellent health mirrors the medical theories that Dr. Wilson believed were most beneficial for women almost forty years ago, in 1966. His theories were based on a patient who had taken estrogen and experienced the advantages of long-term use. Even with all the publicity his book received, the theories were never tested, or at least there is no recorded documentation today available to confirm such an event. However, I wish he were alive today, for I feel that I am the example and product of his theories almost issue for issue. Some people express the belief that hereditary factors and genes are the cause of how good I look and feel today. I am sure that genes, along with my own personal lifestyle, are relevant but as far as the lack of wrinkles, bone loss, mood swings, high energy levels, and the lack of the normal drying out in various feminine areas, research has not discovered that heredity factors and genes have any direct result in those important and specific feminine areas.

<u>Our Womanhood and Spirit</u>

How disheartening to discover that our womanhood and spirit are taken away after giving our best years of our lives to families and careers. Women should have their womanhood protected and maintained throughout their lifetime. They should not ever allow anyone or anything (menopause) to rob them of their womanhood. Men do not lose their masculinity and sex appeal as they proceed through the aging process. Women should expect and demand nothing less. I am sure that people will question my menopause-free existence and the manner in which it was attained, but I believe there is a correlation between my health and my long-term estrogen use. Hopefully, by disclosing my particular case I can bring awareness to everyone that perhaps menopause is really not a necessary part of a woman's life as she enters her later years, just as Dr. Wilson's theory stated.

My thirty-four-year-old daughter told me that she wanted to know *exactly everything* that I have done to maintain my youthfulness, as she wanted to duplicate my method item for item. I did not know at that time that she would not be able to copy my lifestyle. Now more than ever, the importance of sharing my experience has been brought to my attention. I do not know if my situation will make any difference to anyone, especially the medical and pharmaceutical industries, but if I did not at least make an effort to expose what has happened to me, then the lack of effort on my part would have bothered me more than not trying at all. My daughter is now aware of what has happened to me. She does not want any part of menopause, be it the symptoms that take anywhere from five to ten years or the end result, which sadly is the state of taking away womanhood and becoming an old woman. She wants to be just like her mother—a youthful and graceful woman for a lifetime. I am the example of such a medical achievement and women need to know they, too, can possibly achieve the same results!

Putting the Pieces Together

I feel different now that I have put everything together and am at least somewhat able to finally understand why I have never met anyone who is like me. For a while, I actually felt like a fish out of water or an odd person out because so much attention was given to my unusual set of circumstances. The description of me today, as a grandmother of five and sixty-two years old, is that I am 5'3" and weigh approximately 129 pounds. I wear a size four in pants and a medium in tops. I have soft, shiny blonde hair and blue eyes. My legs are very shapely, and I am full of energy. I have maintained my youthful physical appearance, still have my sex appeal and desires, and enjoy lovemaking with my husband of forty-three years. My disposition is positive and harmonious and I have always maintained a positive attitude. I thoroughly enjoy life to its fullest, even when it contains difficulty or tragedy, and I am up to life's challenges and the resolution of all obstacles.

A Cry for Immediate Change

If I have lived my life without as much as one symptom of menopause and without detrimental health changes or the aging process caused by menopause, why can't anyone else? There needs to be a concerted effort made to bring the important health issues of women to the forefront and to have studies and research conducted that will result in favorable changes for women in the areas of today's medical shortcomings. Given today's high standards of medical technology and resources, women should not have to worry about taking drugs that may lead to harmful results or taking drugs that have an unknown future. The entire estrogen environment, which is now very controversial and confusing, is unacceptable. As a result, immediate changes should be forthcoming.

Women deserve and should expect that they, just like men, will have pleasurable, satisfying, and healthy full lives; their enjoyment of life should not be limited to just the first forty-five to fifty years. Let this century be the one that finally brings women medically equal to their counterparts. Perhaps such a result will help to keep marriages, families, and the workplace a happier and more productive environment for all concerned.

The Priorities Once and for All

The number one priority concerning the estrogen environment should be to find out, once and for all, what risks and/or benefits hormones will produce when used long- or short-term. The second priority, given today's standard of living and high-tech capabilities, should be to change, improve, or eliminate the menopause process. The third priority should be to make all of the important information regarding menopause readily available for women so that they can indeed protect their health and be able to make informed medical decisions in a timely manner concerning their important health issues which is impossible for them to do today.

Governed by Chance

I must mention one last important issue concerning my thirty-year usage of estrogen alone. As wonderful as my entire life has been, medically speaking, there is a very large and unsettling factor that needs to be addressed. I live every day of my life not knowing what my future will hold as a result of taking estrogen for thirty years. Will my life continue uneventfully, or will there be drastic and negative results somewhere down the road? There is no way to know the answer, as our medical community has not been able to provide the answer. I have contacted every source with the same questions: What will happen to me? In five years, will I still be as I am today? Will I still be full of energy and experiencing good health? What will happen to me in ten years? Will I ever age in any area? Will I develop cancer at any time in the future? Will I have to take estrogen until the day I die? Will I wake up one day and be wrinkled from head to toe? If I stopped taking estrogen, would my coronary arteries immediately be clogged and cause irreversible heart damage? These are questions that concern me. My health future will always be unknown to me because, as with the rest of the Forgotten Few, that information was not provided in advance of taking estrogen, so my life has always been, and continues to be, governed by chance and the unknown instead of medical knowledge.

After years of questions (including those posed by Dr. Wilson) with no answers, contradictory statements, and opinions, as well as studies, research, and data with no conclusions, accountability, responsibility, and accurate answers must be sought concerning the hormone replacement therapy environment. The medical futures of our young women are deserving and should expect nothing less.

A Major Step in the Right Direction

In an effort to learn more about other long-term estrogen users, I have created a website, www.menopausefree.org, so that 1) long-term estrogen users (more than twenty years) can share their stories and experiences, 2) sufferers, if any, of medical consequences due to the inaccuracy of WHI study results who can share their stories, and 3) signatures can be gathered in an attempt to seek legislation to make it mandatory for all future federally funded estrogen studies to require independent verification *before* announcing the study results. See more details regarding the website on page 150.

Food and Drug Administration (FDA) — Premarin

The estrogen I have been taking for more than thirty years is Premarin. I thought that the history of Premarin, as recorded by the FDA, would be of interest to the public. Therefore, the chart below shows the history of Premarin as being approved by the FDA on May 8, 1942. Please note the section headed **Letters, Reviews, Labels, Patient Package Insert.** Under that heading there was a new dosage regimen change entered on September 8, 1998. That means that Premarin was approved on May 8, 1942 and, other than the new dosage regimen change, 60 years have passed with no other changes or revisions recorded with the FDA until November 27, 2002, which was after the WHI study results were announced.

This is significant information that the general public needs to be aware of for three important reasons: (1) if there had been any negative medical alerts (detrimental health results), 67 years would have been sufficient time for the medical industry to have been given alerts in order to recognize any harm caused by estrogen use; (2) how is it possible that, now, 60 years later, estrogen is now categorized as increasing health risks (when there were no previous alerts); and (3) who is responsible for 67 years of advising women that estrogen use was safe?

These changes, which began in 2002, as shown in the FDA chart below, were a direct result of studies performed starting with the Women's Health Initiative in 2002. It must be remembered the data from that study was misinterpreted in their announcement to the public. However, the most important aspect of study results is this one simple question: *how old were the participants in the studies?* If the participants were *menopausal age and not of the same identical background*, then the chances are great that the study results are subject to question. Again, the mere fact that there were no medical alerts for 60 years is a very a strong statement and one that is difficult to challenge.

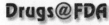

FDA Approved Drug Products

FAQ | Instructions | Glossary | Contact Us | CDER Home

Start Over   Back to Search Results   Back to Overview   Back to Details

Label and Approval History

Drug Name(s)   PREMARIN (Brand Name Drug)

FDA Application No. (NDA) 004782

Active Ingredient(s) ESTROGENS, CONJUGATED

Company   WYETH PHARMS INC

Go to Approval History

Label Information

What information does a label include?
Note: Not all labels are available in electronic format from FDA.

View the label approved on 03/03/2008 🔖 for PREMARIN, NDA no. 004782

- To see older, previously-approved labels, go to the "Approval History" section of this page. **Older labels are for historical information only and should not be used for clinical purposes.**

Approval History
NDA 004782

Note: Not all reviews are available in electronic format from FDA.
Older labels are for historical information only, and should not be used for clinical purposes.
Approval dates can only be verified from 1984 to the present.

Click on a column header to re-sort the table:

Action Date	Supplement Number	Approval Type	Letters, Reviews, Labels, Patient Package Insert	Note
03/03/2008	155	Labeling Revision	Label 🐾 Letter 🔧	
09/05/2006	147	Labeling Revision	Label 🔧 Letter 🔧	
04/24/2006	146	Labeling Revision	Label 🐾 Letter 🔧	
11/01/2005	142	Formulation Revision	Label 🐾 Letter 🔧	
08/01/2005	141	Formulation Revision	Label 🔧 Letter 🔧	
04/07/2005	138	Labeling Revision	Label 🐾 Letter 🔧	
04/07/2005	139	Labeling Revision	Label 🐾 Letter 🔧	
08/26/2004	137	Formulation Revision	Label 🔧 Letter 🔧	
04/20/2004	133	Labeling Revision	Label 🔧 Letter 🔧	
04/20/2004	136	Labeling Revision	Label 🐾 Letter 🔧	
07/16/2003	125	Labeling Revision	Letter 🔧	Label is not available on this site.
04/24/2003	115	New Dosage Regimen	Label 🐾 Letter 🔧 Review 🔧	
04/24/2003	130	Labeling Revision	Label 🐾 Letter 🔧 Review 🔧	
01/07/2003	129	Labeling Revision	Label 🐾 Letter 🔧	
12/20/2002	126	Control Supplement		This supplement type does not usually require new labeling.
11/27/2002	128	Labeling Revision	Label 🔧 Letter 🔧	
08/21/2002	124	Control Supplement		This supplement type does not usually require new labeling.

98

12/03/2001	121	Control Supplement		This supplement type does not usually require new labeling.
08/06/2001	120	Control Supplement		This supplement type does not usually require new labeling.
04/24/2001	116	Expiration Date Change		Label is not available on this site.
07/05/2000	113	Control Supplement		This supplement type does not usually require new labeling.
06/08/1999	109	Labeling Revision		Label is not available on this site.
04/26/1999	086	Control Supplement		This supplement type does not usually require new labeling.
10/29/1998	108	Control Supplement		This supplement type does not usually require new labeling.
09/08/1998	093	New Dosage Regimen	Letter Review	Label is not available on this site.
05/06/1998	096	Labeling Revision		Label is not available on this site.
05/06/1998	104	Labeling Revision		Label is not available on this site.
02/27/1998	101	Control Supplement		This supplement type does not usually require new labeling.
06/28/1996	103	Control Supplement		This supplement type does not usually require new labeling.
06/27/1996	102	Control Supplement		This supplement type does not usually require new labeling.
12/14/1995	100	Control Supplement		This supplement type does not usually require new labeling.
12/13/1995	099	Control Supplement		This supplement type does not usually require new labeling.
04/11/1995	098	Control Supplement		This supplement type does not usually require new labeling.
02/06/1995	095	Manufacturing Change or Addition		This supplement type does not usually require new labeling.
11/09/1994	094	Control Supplement		This supplement type does not usually require new labeling.
12/23/1993	092	Labeling Revision		Label is not available on this site.
03/11/1992	087	Package Change		Label is not available on this site.
05/14/1991	077	Control Supplement		This supplement type does not usually require new labeling.
05/09/1991	078	Expiration Date Change		Label is not available on this site.
02/23/1990	083	Formulation Revision		Label is not available on this site.
12/22/1989	081	Labeling Revision		Label is not available on this site.

05/19/1989	061	Labeling Revision		Label is not available on this site.
05/19/1989	064	Labeling Revision		Label is not available on this site.
05/19/1989	072	Labeling Revision		Label is not available on this site.
05/19/1989	075	Labeling Revision		Label is not available on this site.
05/19/1989	079	Labeling Revision		Label is not available on this site.
02/03/1989	074	Formulation Revision		Label is not available on this site.
12/20/1988	073	Package Change		Label is not available on this site.
04/17/1988	071	Control Supplement		This supplement type does not usually require new labeling.
10/16/1987	068	Control Supplement		This supplement type does not usually require new labeling.
05/14/1987	070	Manufacturing Change or Addition		This supplement type does not usually require new labeling.
12/03/1986	065	Control Supplement		This supplement type does not usually require new labeling.
09/24/1986	066	Manufacturing Change or Addition		This supplement type does not usually require new labeling.
07/10/1986	063	Control Supplement		This supplement type does not usually require new labeling.
05/28/1986	057	Labeling Revision		Label is not available on this site.
05/12/1986	062	Control Supplement		This supplement type does not usually require new labeling.
01/07/1986	060	Formulation Revision		Label is not available on this site.
10/25/1985	059	Package Change		Label is not available on this site.
09/30/1985	058	Control Supplement		This supplement type does not usually require new labeling.
05/29/1985	050	Package Change		Label is not available on this site.
05/29/1985	052	Control Supplement		This supplement type does not usually require new labeling.
04/29/1985	051	Labeling Revision		Label is not available on this site.
04/29/1985	053	Labeling Revision		Label is not available on this site.
04/29/1985	054	Labeling Revision		Label is not available on this site.
01/26/1984	049	Formulation Revision		Label is not available on this site.

05/08/1942	000	Approval		Label is not available on this site.

PDF files, marked with an icon ⤓, require the free <u>Adobe Acrobat Reader</u>.

- **There are no Therapeutic Equivalents**
- <u>**Other Important Information from FDA**</u>

FDA/Center for Drug Evaluation and Research
Office of Training and Communications
Division of Information Services
Update Frequency: Daily

Studying the Wrong Side of the Problem?

Interesting to note, at the beginning of this book in the chapter, *Menopause...In the Beginning*, it is stated that in the early 1800's, once women stopped having their periods, "their diseases increased, including weakness, tumors, cancers and joint pain."

Further, in the chapter, *Dr. Robert A. Wilson*, one of his theories from his 1966 book, *Feminine Forever*, was that "women who were estrogen rich, were cancer poor" and he believed that for maximum health benefits women should remain on estrogen throughout their lives.

Most recently, a study was conducted which revealed that if women have hysterectomies and have their ovaries removed (which eliminates their estrogen production) the risks of dying from all diseases increases, and they will have a significantly higher risk of heart disease, stroke and lung cancer. The study, directed under William H. Parker, M.D., of John Wayne Cancer Institute, raises serious questions about the long-term survival benefits of removing a woman's ovaries during a routine hysterectomy. These results were based on women who had been separated out of the study as a result of not taking hormone replacement therapy after their hysterectomy. Dr. Parker explains that "Before menopause, the ovaries make a lot of estrogen, plus androgens including testosterone and androstenedione. These hormones keep the heart, bones and blood vessels healthy." Further, he explained, "After menopause, the ovaries make less estrogen, but continue to produce androstenedione and testosterone, which are converted by fat and muscle cells into estrogen. So there is a continued source of estrogen from these hormones that continues to protect the blood vessels. If you remove the ovaries, you lose the estrogen and the androgens, and the benefits to the blood vessels."

Think about what that study said — it states clearly that estrogen is needed to keep the heart, bones and blood vessels healthy. Logically thinking, when menopause occurs and the estrogen is decreased — what would happen to those important organs if they got a boost of estrogen by choice — or even better, the estrogen was never decreased?

"Nobody to date had thought to look at the big picture," Dr. Parker said. "That is, how does the survival data actually inform the decision about whether to take out the ovaries or not?" Put in simple terms, that statement raises the question of how important are the ovaries and the estrogen they produce?

Those are very important results. However, it is more interesting to note that no studies or research have been conducted to see if maintaining estrogen prevents disease and cancer. Most of the studies and research are conducted on women around the age of menopause, which is fifty-one. What if maintaining estrogen lifelong is actually the answer? How does anyone know if the theory has not been studied, researched or tested? Once again, as I have presently stated, there are millions of long-term estrogen users. I wonder what their lives have been like? Perhaps it's time to try to get an idea of their outcomes.

Because of my mother's hysterectomy at such a young age, her body was without estrogen for forty-two years. She contracted pancreatic cancer at age sixty-six. No one in the family has ever had any form of cancer. Such a theory definitely gains my attention. Under such a hypothesis, for women who have an early menopause, say, in her early to middle forties, and lose their estrogen production, does that mean twenty years later, at age sixty-two or so, that the risk factor of early loss of estrogen will increase their chances of contracting cancer? Of course, there is no way of knowing, but if three previous references have indicated such a possibility, perhaps it is not estrogen being given at the menopausal age of fifty that creates the damage, but the *opposite* — NOT having estrogen for twenty years — that creates the damage.

Estrogen usage, to date, has no concrete risk or benefit conclusion. Apparently, the main concern is, once again, the menopausal women — lowest dosage for the shortest period of time. Maybe it's time to study the entire environment — youth (twenties and thirties, with estrogen) and the older women (forties and fifties, decreasing estrogen). What is the difference in those two groups of women and their health? What makes the twenty and thirty-year-old women healthy and vibrant versus the forty and fifty-year-old women who have started losing their health and energy?

It is time that the entire estrogen environment be studied and not just half of it. Let's find out what makes us healthy in our youth and apply it to our aging years. Waiting until age fifty is too late. Any hereditary factors or predisposed health factors would already be in place. In other words, at age fifty, the harm has already started.

Breast Cancer and Estrogen

Dr. Crandall

Breast cancer is the most common cancer of nonsmoking women and the second most common cancer of smoking women. One in eight women will develop breast cancer in her lifetime. Not taking estrogen will not decrease the risk of developing breast cancer. This is demonstrated by the progressive increase in the diagnosis of breast cancer with age in the WHI CEE plus MPA study. This is the cumulative incidence of breast cancer in the women who are not taking estrogen. When do they stop getting more?

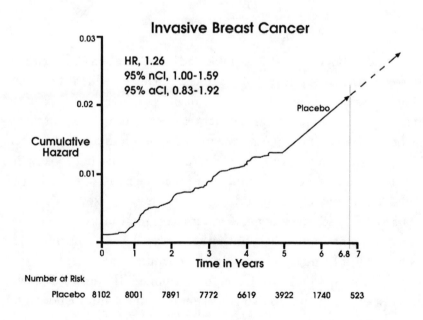

This is a total of 124 cases of breast cancer in 8,102 women who never took estrogen. Very similar results are seen in a collaborative series[14] of 12,467 cases of breast cancer in never-users of estrogen.

Estimated cumulative number of breast cancers diagnosed in 1000 never-users of HRT.

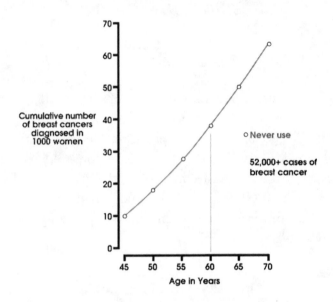

The collaborative study was published in 1997 in *Lancet*. The authors looked at the five- and ten-year marks and concluded that hormones should be stopped because of a "statistically significant" increase in the number of cases of breast cancer after ten years of use. Instead of thirty-eight cases per one thousand women in the non-hormone users, there were forty-two cases in the hormone users. They did not look at the development of cancer over time to see that the non-users also had 42 cases at ten years eleven months. In a disease that takes seven to ten years to diagnose, this study does not indicate more breast cancer at ten years in the hormone users, but rather *earlier diagnosis!* In this study, as in the WHI study, the question is, when do women get less breast cancer if they do not take estrogen or hormones? The answer is, never! It is just diagnosed one to two years later in women who are not taking hormones.

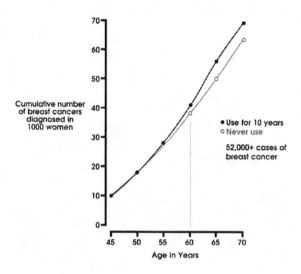

Estimated cumulative number of breast cancers diagnosed in
1000 never-users of HRT and 1000 users of HRT for 10 years.

To understand the effect of hormones on this progressive increase
in breast cancer throughout a woman's life, it is important to review the
natural history of breast cancer. In the figure[10,11] below, you see that the
time it takes for a tumor to progress from a single cancer cell to a size
large enough to show on a mammogram is just less than seven years. It
takes another three years before it is large enough to palpate. This is very
important when evaluating the WHI data about breast cancer. In the
WHI, the average size of breast cancers diagnosed was 1.5cm.

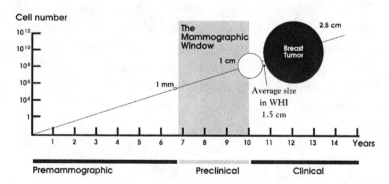

There are no new breast cancers,
they were there when the study started!

107

The next area to examine is the incidence of breast cancer over time in women on estrogen. The graph below from the WHI[3] shows that women on estrogen alone (CEE) actually had fewer breast cancers than women on a placebo. This was ignored by the news media and the WHI. Apparently good news is no news.

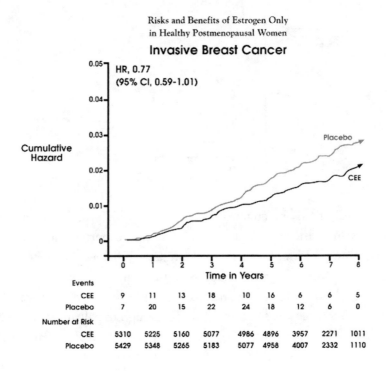

Risks and Benefits of Estrogen Only
in Healthy Postmenopausal Women

Invasive Breast Cancer

HR, 0.77
(95% CI, 0.59-1.01)

Events									
CEE	9	11	13	18	10	16	6	6	5
Placebo	7	20	15	22	24	18	12	6	0
Number at Risk									
CEE	5310	5225	5160	5077	4986	4896	3957	2271	1011
Placebo	5429	5348	5265	5183	5077	4958	4007	2332	1110

The mass hysteria created by the news media was caused by the misunderstanding of the following graph[2] of the incidence of breast cancer in women on placebo or on estrogen plus progestin. Remember that it takes seven to ten years before breast cancer can be diagnosed from the first cancer cell and that the average woman was in this study for only 5.6 years.

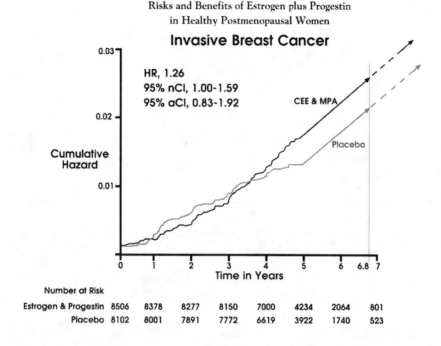

Risks and Benefits of Estrogen plus Progestin
in Healthy Postmenopausal Women

Invasive Breast Cancer

HR, 1.26
95% nCI, 1.00-1.59
95% aCI, 0.83-1.92

CEE & MPA

Placebo

Cumulative
Hazard

Time in Years

0.03
0.02
0.01

0   1   2   3   4   5   6 6.8 7

Number at Risk

Estrogen & Progestin	8506	8378	8277	8150	7000	4234	2064	801
Placebo	8102	8001	7891	7772	6619	3922	1740	523

Taking into account the length of time women were in the study (5.6 years) and the length of time it takes to diagnose breast cancer (seven to ten years) it is obvious that there were no new breast cancers. All the breast cancers were present when the study started! There were a few breast cancers that grew rapidly in the presence of estrogen and progestin and were found earlier in the fifth year, but the onset of diagnosis of breast cancer is the same in both groups after that.

Logic would suggest that if breast cancer is diagnosed earlier, a better prognosis is expected. A review[7] of the relative risk of mortality from breast cancer when on estrogen was published, and it reveals that most studies showed a decreased risk of dying from breast cancer with hormone use. The next figure[7] from that study shows the results of multiple studies evaluating this.

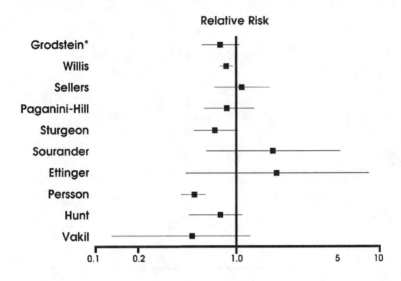

Risk of Dying from Breast Cancer with Hormone Use
*current use

This graph shows the results from multiple studies. The small square is the relative risk. The bar shows the confidence interval (CI) for that study. The narrower the confidence interval, the more certain the results. If the confidence interval does not cross 1.0, then the results are "statistically significant." The two most certain studies are also the only statistically significant studies. One shows about a 10 percent decrease and the other a 40 percent decrease in the relative risk of dying from breast cancer with hormone use at the time of diagnosis. Four other studies show a nonsignificant decrease in the risk, but if these studies were only a little more certain, they would also show a significant decrease.

In summary, women who do not take estrogen and progestin have just as many occurrences of breast cancer within a few months to two years and worse prognoses when they are diagnosed with breast cancer as those who do take estrogen and progestin. If a woman truly wants to decrease her risk of dying from breast cancer, she should take estrogen so if she develops cancer, it will be identified earlier and have a better prognosis.

Cumulative summary:

1. The WHI ignored the natural history of breast cancer.

2. Breast cancer is diagnosed earlier in women who take estrogen and progestin. Women who do not take estrogen are diagnosed with breast cancer just as often as those who do within one to two years.

3. In the WHI studies, there was no new breast cancer.

4. The risk of dying from breast cancer is decreased in women taking hormones according to most studies published.

Heart Attacks

Heart attacks are the most common cause of death in men and women.[9] The natural history of a heart attack takes fifteen to twenty years to develop.[12] It starts with a cholesterol deposit that grows over time, narrowing the coronary artery. Ultimately, the cholesterol calcifies and becomes fragile. Finally, the surface cracks and becomes rough, and a clot (thrombosis) forms on the cholesterol plaque, suddenly blocking the artery. This is known as an acute coronary thrombosis, or heart attack. Observational studies have shown for years that women on hormones in menopause have fewer heart attacks than women not on hormones.[15,16,17] In addition, when young women have their ovaries removed and do not take estrogen, their risk of a heart attack rapidly becomes equal to that of a man of the same age.[18] This was interpreted by some to mean that estrogen or other hormones should prevent heart attacks in all risk groups.

The HERS[19] study in 1998 was designed to examine this. Women who were at high risk for heart attacks were recruited to start oral conjugated equine estrogen plus progestin or a placebo to prevent another heart attack. The HERS II[20] study followed up on the original study and found that women who were at risk for heart attacks continued to have more heart attacks (Imagine that!). Apparently the researchers forgot that oral CEE plus progestin induces clotting factors and that a heart attack is a clotting event at an area of roughened cholesterol plaque in a coronary artery. Fortunately, the results were not worse. As one would expect, there were more heart attacks in the CEE plus progestin group, but in less than one year the women in the placebo group had just as many clotting events in the hearts (heart attacks). The graph below is from the HERS II study; the HERS study only included the first five years.

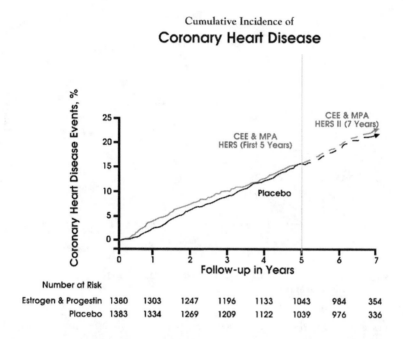

Cumulative Incidence of
Coronary Heart Disease

Number at Risk								
Estrogen & Progestin	1380	1303	1247	1196	1133	1043	984	354
Placebo	1383	1334	1269	1209	1122	1039	976	336

No one ever claimed that giving oral clot-inducing hormones to someone who was at risk for a clotting event would decrease their risk of a clotting event. These results were seized upon hysterically to prove that taking estrogen does not prevent heart attacks. It only shows that the pathophysiology of diseases and the pharmacology of hormones or treatments should be known before studies are designed or interpreted.

The WHI started over 16,000 women on either oral CEE plus MPA or a placebo in a randomized but clinically unblind fashion. These women were very well randomized in regard to multiple risk factors. It is easy to assume that an equal number in each group were about to have a heart attack (acute coronary thrombosis). This risk had been developing over the last fifteen to twenty years because of their lifestyles, genetics, and environments. The graph below shows the results.

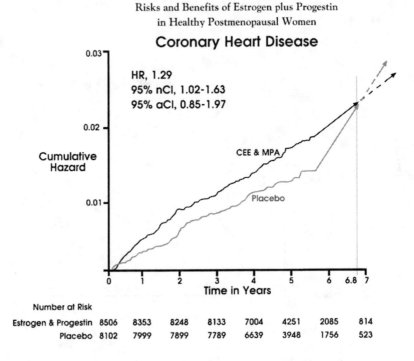

Risks and Benefits of Estrogen plus Progestin
in Healthy Postmenopausal Women

Coronary Heart Disease

HR, 1.29
95% nCI, 1.02-1.63
95% aCI, 0.85-1.97

Cumulative Hazard

CEE & MPA

Placebo

Time in Years

Number at Risk								
Estrogen & Progestin	8506	8353	8248	8133	7004	4251	2085	814
Placebo	8102	7999	7899	7789	6639	3948	1756	523

As expected, there were more heart attacks in the first year in the CEE+MPA group. However, the placebo group caught up the next year, and for the next five years the rates increased similarly. In the sixth year, there is a rapid rise in the number of heart attacks in the placebo group, and if the graphs are extrapolated, the placebo group will pass the CEE+MPA group at seven years. Taking into account the natural history of heart attacks, this is sooner than expected. Because it takes fifteen years for a heart attack to develop, you would expect that it would take fifteen years to see any benefit from hormone usage. Very similar results are seen in the WHI CEE only group in the graph below. Interestingly, there are no differences until the sixth year, when the placebo group begins to have more heart attacks.

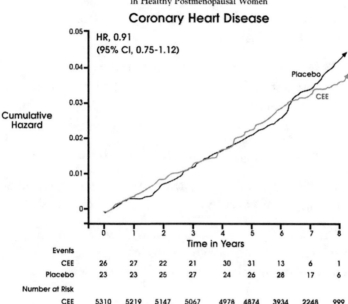

Risks and Benefits of Estrogen Only
in Healthy Postmenopausal Women

Coronary Heart Disease

HR, 0.91
(95% CI, 0.75-1.12)

Cumulative Hazard

Placebo

CEE

Time in Years

Events									
CEE	26	27	22	21	30	31	13	6	1
Placebo	23	23	25	27	24	26	28	17	6
Number at Risk									
CEE	5310	5219	5147	5067	4978	4874	3934	2248	999
Placebo	5429	5336	5254	5171	5072	4959	4015	2331	1106

The bottom line is that taking hormones does not increase the risk of a heart attack. Poor prescribing increases the risk of a heart attack if one is ready to happen. Oral hormones should not be prescribed if there is a risk of a heart attack or a history of a prior heart attack. Women who have had a heart attack should switch to transdermal estrogen or estrogen and a progestin. Women should stop taking estrogen or hormones after a heart attack as often as men are castrated to prevent heart attacks. That, of course, means *never!* Stopping the use of estrogen or hormones after a heart attack can lead to vascular instability and coronary spasms, thereby increasing the risk of a new heart attack.[21] After a heart attack, women should continue the use of or change to transdermal or transvaginal hormones. If there are risk factors for coronary artery disease, then oral estrogen or progestins usually should not be used. Risk factors include tobacco use, prior tobacco use, high blood pressure, high cholesterol, diabetes, more than two years without hormones or a strong family history of heart disease. These are relative, non-absolute reasons to switch to non-oral hormones.

Cumulative summary:

1. The WHI ignored the natural history of breast cancer and heart disease.

2. Breast cancer is diagnosed earlier in women who take estrogen and progestin. Women who do not take estrogen are diagnosed with breast cancer just as often as those who do within one to two years.

3. In the WHI studies, there was no new breast cancer.

4. The risk of dying from breast cancer is decreased in women taking hormones according to most studies published.

5. The WHI ignored the pharmacology of conjugated equine estrogen and medroxyprogesterone acetate and the relative reasons not to take them orally.

6. Heart disease is decreased if hormones are begun at menopause and continued for life.

7. Women with risk factors for heart disease should use transdermal or transvaginal estrogen (and progestin if needed).

8. Cardiac benefits of restarting estrogen should not be expected for fifteen years based on the natural history of heart attacks.

Hip Fracture

Estrogen is needed for normal functioning of almost all tissues in the body. One tissue that can be measured to show the effects of estrogen deficiency is bone. The weakening of bone is called osteoporosis. A measure of osteoporosis is hip fracture rate. Despite what the WHI and NIH would want women to believe, women do not get just osteoporosis when they are estrogen deficient; they get "body-porosis." Most tissues atrophy, wither, and become "porotic" without estrogen. There is a lot more to women than their bones. Examining the WHI hip fracture graph from the CEE+MPA study reveals some frightening information.

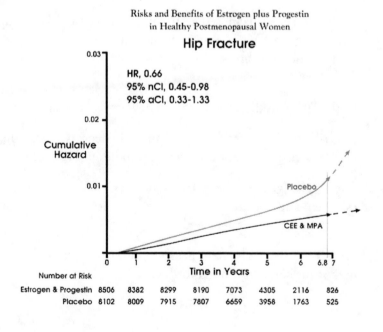

Risks and Benefits of Estrogen plus Progestin
in Healthy Postmenopausal Women

Hip Fracture

HR, 0.66
95% nCI, 0.45-0.98
95% aCI, 0.33-1.33

Cumulative Hazard

Placebo

CEE & MPA

Time in Years

Number at Risk	0	1	2	3	4	5	6	6.8
Estrogen & Progestin	8506	8382	8299	8190	7073	4305	2116	826
Placebo	8102	8009	7915	7807	6659	3958	1763	525

There is a gradual increase in the number of fractures in the placebo group until the sixth year, and then a rapid increase in the fracture rate in the placebo group occurs. In the CEE+MPA study, there is a leveling off of the fracture rate in the hormone users, showing a true preventive effect. The most disturbing thing about this graph is the pain, disability, and prognosis associated with a hip fracture. *The Textbook of Orthopedics*[22] states a 15 to 20 percent mortality rate in the first six months after hip fracture; 25 percent of the patients will never walk independently again, and the rest will recover after major surgery and prolonged physical therapy. Compare this to early-stage breast cancer in women on hormones (Grade 1, Stage 1, Estrogen receptor and Progesterone receptor positive), which has a 98 percent cure rate[23]. Most women who have known family or friends with both would not choose to have hip fracture over breast cancer. Remember, though, that not taking estrogen does not reduce the risk of getting breast cancer. It only delays the diagnosis and worsens the prognosis.

Cumulative summary:

1. The WHI ignored the natural history of breast cancer and heart disease.

2. Breast cancer is diagnosed earlier in women who take estrogen and progestin. Women who do not take estrogen are just as likely to develop breast cancer as those who do within one to two years.

3. In the WHI studies, there was no new breast cancer.

4. The risk of dying from breast cancer is decreased in women taking hormones according to most studies published.

5. The WHI ignored the pharmacology of conjugated equine estrogen and medroxyprogesterone acetate and the relative reasons not to take them orally.

6. The risk of heart disease is decreased if hormones are begun at menopause and continued for life.

7. Women with risk factors for heart disease should use transdermal or transvaginal estrogen (and progestin if needed).

8. Cardiac benefits of restarting estrogen should not be expected for fifteen years based on the natural history of heart attacks.

9. Hormones reduce the risk of hip and other fractures. Hip fracture is much more painful and debilitating, and has a worse prognosis, than breast cancer.

Alzheimer's Disease

Alzheimer's disease is a progressive loss of brain function due to progressive destruction of the brain by a poorly understood process. It has been shown that starting the use of estrogen after the development of Alzheimer's disease has no effect on the progression or prognosis.[24,25,26] This is expected if you realize that by the time symptoms appear, there is usually significant microscopic damage to the nerve cells in the brain. Alzheimer's disease is predominantly a disease of women. Three women will develop Alzheimer's disease for every man.[27] Seventy-one percent of nursing home occupants are women. Multiple observational studies have been done to determine the effect on the risk of Alzheimer's disease when women take estrogen.[4,5,6] Eleven of these studies are in the graph[4] below.

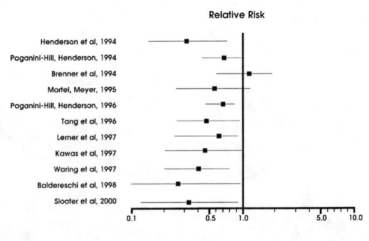

Risk of Alzheimer''s Disease

This graph also depicts the relative risk as a small square with confidence intervals surrounding each risk. Seven of these studies show a significant reduction from 20 to 75 percent in the risk of Alzheimer's disease when women take estrogen. Three studies also show a non-significant decrease in the risk of Alzheimer's disease with estrogen use. One study is neutral. If any treatment for men showed such an incredibly positive benefit, there would probably be a public service announcement between each quarter of all broadcast football games and in every edition of *Sports Illustrated* telling viewers to use that treatment.

The prognosis for Alzheimer's disease is horrible.[28] The graph below shows the survival curve for patients with probable Alzheimer's disease, possible Alzheimer's disease, and vascular dementia. It is the same for all three.

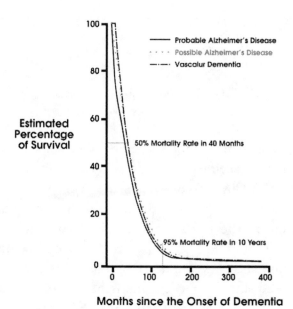

Months since the Onset of Dementia

The most shocking thing is the 50 percent mortality at forty months (three years four months) and the approximate 95 percent mortality at 120 months (ten years). Compare this to the 98 percent five-year survival for localized breast cancer and the 88 percent five-year survival for all new cases of breast cancer.[23]

Another study was published after the first WHI paper on the risk of Alzheimer's disease in women and men in Cache County, Utah.[6] The results of this study agree with the other studies published and with reality. The results are below in a graphical form.

Hormone Replacement Therapy and Incidence of
Alzheimer's Disease in Older Women

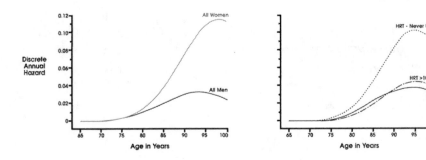

Estimated Discrete Yearly Risk of Alzheimer's Disease for Men and Women by Age
and by Duration of Hormone Replacement

The first thing to note in the left graph is that women have a higher risk of developing Alzheimer's disease than men. In the right graph, the women are separated by years of estrogen use. Women on hormones for longer than ten years had one-fourth the risk of developing Alzheimer's disease of women who never took hormones! Although women on hormones for a shorter time had a lower risk of developing Alzheimer's, it was not significantly lower until ten or more years of use.

One of the explanations for dementia is the observation that estrogen is necessary for glucose transport across the blood-brain barrier.[29] The blood-brain barrier is a membrane in the brain between the blood in the blood vessel or capillary and the brain tissue. Many nutrients have to be actively transported across the blood-brain barrier to get to the brain. Most tissues in the body can live on various simple sugars, fats, or amino acids. The brain, however, requires glucose to make energy and stay healthy. Without estrogen, the blood-brain barrier is unable to transport enough glucose to keep the brain cells well fed. The starving brain cells send out a signal telling the body to make more glucose, which is part of what happens during a hot flash. Unfortunately, as hot flashes continue, the blood-brain barrier cannot transport glucose into the brain, and the brain starves. Eventually, the part of the brain that senses the lack of glucose and sends the signal dies, and the hot flashes stop. In some women whose hot flashes have stopped after low doses of estrogen have been initiated, hot flashes resume until physiologic levels of estrogen are reached.[30] Apparently, the starvation sensing part of the brain has not died in these cases; it has just gone dormant. Hot flashes and night sweats that are due to estrogen deficiency are not funny or something to joke about. These symptoms are signaling brain starvation and need to be stopped. A patient once asked, "Why would I have such a horrible symptom if something was not horribly wrong?"

Cumulative summary:

1. The WHI ignored the natural history of breast cancer and heart disease.

2. Breast cancer is diagnosed earlier in women who take estrogen and progestin. Women who do not take estrogen are just as likely to develop breast cancer as those who do within one to two years.

3. In the WHI studies, there was no new breast cancer.

4. The risk of dying from breast cancer is decreased in women taking hormones according to most studies published.

5. The WHI ignored the pharmacology of conjugated equine estrogen and medroxyprogesterone acetate and the relative reasons not to take them orally.

6. The risk of heart disease is decreased if hormones are begun at menopause and continued for life.

7. Women with risk factors for heart disease should use transdermal or transvaginal estrogen (and progestin if needed).

8. Cardiac benefits of restarting estrogen should not be expected for fifteen years based on the natural history of heart attacks.

9. Hormones reduce the risk of hip and other fractures. Hip fracture is much more painful and debilitating, and has a worse prognosis, than breast cancer.

10. The risk of Alzheimer's disease is significantly reduced with estrogen use.

11. The risk of nursing home placement (loss of independence) is significantly reduced with estrogen use.

12. Hot flashes are a symptom of the brain starving and should be stopped with estrogen replacement if possible.

WHIMS Study

The Women's Health Initiative Memory Study[31,32,33] was designed to examine the effect of conjugated equine estrogen (CEE) plus progestin (MPA) and the effect of CEE alone on cognitive function in postmenopausal women. The women in the study had to be age sixty-five or older, and hot flashes had to have been resolved prior to entering the WHI studies. Two studies were performed: the CEE plus MPA and the CEE alone. Pooled results were published in the CEE-alone report. Women were certified as free of dementia by a standard protocol. Unfortunately, the designers did not show that the women were free of cerebrovascular disease (hardening of the arteries in the brain), and they apparently ignored or were unaware that oral CEE and MPA induce clotting factors as they pass through the liver. In all, 45 percent of the women were smokers or ex-smokers, 55 percent had hypertension, and 10 percent were diabetic. All of these are risk factors for hardening of the arteries and small vessel disease in the brain. Progression of pre-existing cerebrovascular disease when clotting factors are suddenly increased is not a surprise. Thankfully, there were no more problems. The conclusions were that CEE causes a decrease in cognition and causes the onset of dementia. The conclusion should have been: Do not prescribe full-strength oral hormones that induce clotting factors to women with pre-existing vascular disease in the brain, and understand the natural history of diseases before studying them.

There is overwhelming observational evidence from multiple studies indicating that women who take estrogen for longer than ten years experience a significant reduction in the incidence of dementia.[4,5,6] Indeed, a woman's risk of Alzheimer's disease is reduced to the same risk as that of a man if she takes estrogen throughout her life.[6] Her risk of Alzheimer's, when taking appropriate amounts of estrogen, is one-fourth of what it would be if she took no estrogen.[5,6] This dichotomy of conclusions points out that if conclusions (such as those of the WHI and WHIMS) do not agree with most prior studies, outside consultation with someone who understands the diseases studied and the treatments used should be sought. The conclusion that all prior observational studies are incorrect because the newest study disagrees is arrogant and dangerous.

Pre-Mature Mortality

Death is significantly reduced in women taking estrogen or hormones. A study looking at mortality in women on estrogen in the Kaiser Permanente group was published in 1996.[34] The graph below illustrates the percentages of women surviving in both groups.

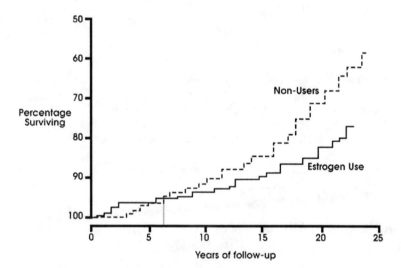

All-cause mortality in postmenopausal women using estrogen versus that in matched controls

This was a twenty-three-year study. It is interesting to note that in the first seven years, there were more deaths in the estrogen group. Not surprisingly, the first seven years parallels the coronary heart disease graph from the WHI CEE plus MPA study. When this study was begun, there was only oral estrogen available, and a few women were taking monthly injections. After the seventh year, however, the number of deaths in the nonuser group steadily pulls away. In the twenty-third year, 80 percent of the estrogen users were alive and 60 percent of the nonusers were alive. In the United States, there are 40 million postmenopausal women. Extrapolating this result to all 40 million women gives a figure of 8 million excess deaths of women in twenty-three years if they do not take estrogen. If all postmenopausal women in the world do not take estrogen, there will be over 100 million excess deaths over the next twenty-three years.

The Nurses' Health Study also published a mortality paper in 1997.[35] This was a much larger study involving over 10,000 women. Mortality was analyzed over eighteen years. The results are summarized below:

Reduction of Risk of Death for Women on Hormones

		Confidence Interval (CI)
All Causes of Death	37% Decreased	(33% to 44%)
Heart Attack Deaths	53% Decreased	(31% to 68%)
All Cancer Deaths	29% Decreased	(19% to 38%
Breast Cancer Deaths	24% Decreased	(-2% to 44%)

(The study is not quite significant because the CI crosses zero, but it agrees with most other studies.)

Reduction in All-Cause Mortality on Hormones for Various Risk Groups

Risk Factor	Decrease in All-Cause Mortality	CI
High Cardiovascular Risk	49% Decrease	(43% to 55%)
Breast Cancer in Mother or Sister	35% Decrease	(10% to 53%)
Age 50 to 59	37% Decrease	(27% to 47%)
Age 60 to 73	42% Decrease	(32% to 51%)

Less than 50 at Menopause	42% Decrease	(30% to 52%)
Older than 53 at Menopause	38% Decrease	(3% to 61%)
Smoker	45% Decrease	(33% to 55%)
Never a Smoker	36% Decrease	(33% to 47%)
Surgical Menopause	29% Decrease	(7% to 45%)
Natural Menopause	41% Decrease	(32% to 49%)
Thin	37% Decrease	(26 to 47%)
Obese	46% Decrease	(28 to 59%).

The risk of dying was decreased in all risk groups! It was never increased!

The question is: When is it bad to take hormones?

The answer is, almost never!

Cumulative summary:

1. The WHI ignored the natural history of breast cancer and heart disease.

2. Breast cancer is diagnosed earlier in women who take estrogen and progestin. Women who do not take estrogen are just as likely to develop breast cancer as those who do within one to two years.

3. In the WHI studies, there was no new breast cancer.

4. The risk of dying from breast cancer is decreased in women taking hormones according to most studies published.

5. The WHI ignored the pharmacology of conjugated equine estrogen and medroxyprogesterone acetate and the relative reasons not to take them orally.

6. The risk of heart disease is decreased if hormones are begun at menopause and continued for life.

7. Women with risk factors for heart disease should use transdermal or transvaginal estrogen (and progestin if needed).

8. Cardiac benefits of restarting estrogen should not be expected for fifteen years based on the natural history of heart attacks.

9. Hormones reduce the risk of hip and other fractures. Hip fracture is much more painful and debilitating, and has a worse prognosis, than breast cancer.

10. The risk of Alzheimer's disease is significantly reduced with estrogen use.

11. The risk of nursing home placement (loss of independence) is significantly reduced with estrogen use.

12. Hot flashes are a symptom of the brain starving and should be stopped with estrogen replacement if possible.

13. Estrogen decreases the risk of death from all causes by 33 to 37%.

14. The risk of dying from a heart attack is reduced by 53% with estrogen use.

15. The risk of dying from all cancers is reduced by 29% with estrogen use.

16. Women with a mother or sister with breast cancer will experience a 35% reduction in dying from all causes with estrogen use.

17. Women in all risk groups will experience a significant reduction in the risk of dying with estrogen use.

Hormone Replacement

Understanding estrogen replacement requires an understanding of the natural cycle of estrogen and progesterone in a pre-menopausal woman. The cycling of estrogen and progesterone prepares the uterus and the body for pregnancy each month. In a normal cycle,36 the estradiol level is 40 pg/ml during days one to four of the cycle, and the level rises to 50 pg/ml on day five of the cycle. Over the next five days, the level rises to 100 pg/ml. The estradiol level rises rapidly over the next two days to about 400 pg/ml. Over the next two days it falls back to about 100 pg/ml, and then it rises to about 250pg/ml from days sixteen to twenty-six of the cycle. It then rapidly falls back to 40 pg/ml to begin the next cycle. The goal of estrogen replacement is to achieve a continuous level of 50 pg/ml to 150 pg/ml (like day five through day ten of a normal cycle) to relieve estrogen deficiency symptoms and prevent symptoms caused by the presence of too much estrogen. Some women will need to have levels of 100 pg/ml to 180 pg/ml for the relief of symptoms, and for some a level above 49 pg/ml will be too much. Each woman is different. No one replacement level or regimen will be right for every woman. I will try to review most common situations.

Surgical Menopause

Donna went through surgical menopause over thirty years ago. She was placed on Premarin (conjugated equine estrogen) because that was the only available oral estrogen replacement at that time. This was the first oral estrogen available, and it has been taken by tens of millions of women. Donna is having no problems with Premarin; she has no reason to stop now, and she should continue the Premarin for the rest of her life. *Donna is correct in her assumption that the amazing state of her health is attributable to the Premarin.* The NIH, WHI, FDA, and her doctors want her to stop taking it to reduce her risk of breast cancer, heart attack, stroke, and blood clots in her legs and lungs. As you will recall, women not taking estrogen had the same amount of breast cancer as the estrogen users in all studies. If she was going to have blood clots, she already would have had blood clots years ago. Stopping Premarin would significantly worsen her health, not improve it. Women on Premarin who are doing well should continue it for the rest of their lives unless medical conditions develop that are reasons for them to switch to transdermal or transvaginal estrogen. Women should not stop taking estrogen if they have a heart attack, stroke, transient ischemic attack (TIA), or deep vein thrombosis (DVT). Women should only stop taking estrogen for the same reasons the doctor would recommend castration for a man with the same condition. Switching from an oral to a transdermal or transvaginal form of estrogen would be appropriate, but stopping the estrogen would not. There are some rare clotting disorders that women and men develop that any type or dose of sex hormones seem to make worse.

Women who have gone through surgical menopause and women who have had a hysterectomy prior to menopause who enter menopause naturally both need only estrogen replacement. There are many new options for estrogen replacement for postmenopausal women.

There are many different ways to replace estradiol (bioidentical estrogen). The following is a list of most of the available replacements:

Pills Femtrace (estradiol acetate)
   Estrace, Gynodiol (micronized bioidentical estradiol)
   Micronized bioidentical estradiol generic
   Premarin (conjugated equine estrogen)
   Cenestin (synthetic conjugated equine estrogen)
   Ogen, Orthoest (estropipate) (estrone)
Transdermal Patches (all provide bioidentical estradiol)
   Alora (once weekly bioidentical estradiol)
   Climara (once weekly bioidentical estradiol)
   Esclim (twice weekly bioidentical estradiol)
   Estraderm (twice weekly bioidentical estradiol)
   FemPatch (once weekly bioidentical estradiol)
   Vivelle (twice weekly bioidentical estradiol)
   Vivelle Dot (twice weekly bioidentical estradiol)
Transdermal Gel
   Divigel (bioidentical estradiol)
   Estrogel (bioidentical estradiol)
   Elestrin (bioidentical estradiol)
Transdermal Lotion
   Estrasorb (bioidentical estradiol)
Transvaginal Ring
   Femring (bioidentical estradiol)
Vaginal Tablet (local effect only)
   Vagifem Tablets (bioidentical estradiol)
Vaginal Ring (local effect only)
   Estring (bioidentical estradiol)
Vaginal Creams
   Estrace Cream (bioidentical estradiol)
   Premarin Cream (CEE)

There are a large number of choices for estrogen-only replacement. The first choice is method of delivery: transdermal, transvaginal, or oral. Oral replacement would be appropriate for someone who had taken birth control pills without problems and is just starting menopause. Oral hormones are absorbed in the stomach or small intestine and pass through the liver first. This passage through the liver induces clotting, diabetes, migraines, and high-blood-pressure factors. This makes any risk factors for heart attack, stroke, blood clots in the legs, smoking, diabetes, migraine headaches, and high blood pressure relative reasons to not take oral hormones. Some women, however, prefer to take oral hormones and would rather accept the very small risk associated with taking oral hormones than use another type of estrogen. Generic oral bioidentical estradiol is the least expensive of all estrogen replacements at four dollars for one month or ten dollars for three months of estrogen replacement.

Transdermal patches have the advantage of being available in multiple dosage levels and brands. Generic estradiol patches have failed to deliver consistent levels of estrogen or stick to the skin well. Generic substitution is not acceptable with estradiol patches. The patch chosen should be one that has multiple doses and is available in local pharmacies. The favorite one-week patch seems to be Climara, and the favorite twice-weekly patch is the Vivelle Dot. The Vivelle Dot is the only patch with no generic "equivalent". This helps the consumer avoid "discussions" involving pharmacies and drug plans. Vivelle Dot is also the smallest of all the patches and is found in most pharmacies.

Transdermal bioidentical estradiol gels are Divigel, Estrogel and Elestrin. Many women prefer gels, but they come in a strength that is too weak for many women. The FDA unquestioningly accepted the conclusions of the WHI and thinks that women should take a low or inadequate dose of estrogen for five years or less. With hope, when the inaccuracy of the WHI is realized the FDA will encourage lifelong physiologic gel replacement by making stronger gels available to women who need them. Estragel and Elestrin come in a pump, and dosing is limited to one to three pumps daily. Three pumps can be used, but this empties the bottle quickly.

There is one transdermal bioidentical estradiol lotion—Estrasorb, which is available commercially. It comes in small packets. The usual dose is one or two packets daily, with most women requiring two packets daily. It is not strong enough for many young women. There are many compounded lotions and creams available. "Experts" have criticized these because the FDA does not control them. Just like commercial products, these products require estradiol level tests to get the concentration at a therapeutic level for the woman. Women are very different in their absorption and metabolism of estradiol no matter how it is given. Compounded lotions and creams have been found to contain much more consistent levels of estradiol than generic estradiol patches. The disadvantage is they have to be compounded at "compounding" pharmacies, which are not as convenient as the large chain pharmacies. The cost of compounded lotions and creams can vary much more than that of commercial products; again, this depends on the pharmacy.

Evamist is a bioidentical estradiol spray. One to three sprays are used daily on the forearm, lower abdomen, thighs or buttocks. The spray dries quickly and the estradiol is absorbed throughout the day.

The transvaginal bioidentical estradiol ring, Femring, is one of the latest delivery methods. It only comes in two strengths, but it is an excellent choice for many women. The Femring's advantage is that it lasts three months. It also provides a very stable level of estrogen, which can reduce the number of migraines in women whose migraines are worsened by changes in hormone levels. Most women and their partners do not notice the transvaginal ring when it has been properly placed. It fits like the ring of a diaphragm. A small number of couples (less than 5 percent) remove the ring for intercourse and replace it afterwards. The risk of yeast or bacterial vaginal infections is actually decreased in women using the Femring, as the high level of estrogen it creates in the vagina makes the vaginal lining thicken and lowers the pH in the vagina. This encourages the growth of healthy vaginal bacteria and discourages the growth of yeast and "bad" bacteria.

Vaginal creams have been available for years and have been sold to improve vaginal health in women who should not or choose not to take estrogen systemically. Before the first patch, Estraderm, was available,

Estrace cream (bioidentical estradiol) could be used in very small doses to achieve excellent estradiol levels in women intravaginally. If a vaginal applicator is used to place cream in the vagina, the cream has to be viewed as a systemic, not a topical, treatment. They are only local topical therapies if they are rubbed into the tissues in small amounts. They are excellent choices for initiating treatment of atrophic vaginitis to speed the recovery of the vagina from estrogen deficiency. The vaginal cream should be stopped one week before estradiol levels are checked to accurately reflect the amount of systemic estradiol. The quality of Generic estradiol vaginal creams has been found to be inconsistent, and I cannot recommend them.

The bioidentical estradiol vaginal tablet Vagifem is preferred by many women because they do not like inserting cream and because the cream will occasionally come out after insertion. The other advantage is that the tablets can be used twice weekly with excellent results. The estradiol is in a bioadhesive tablet that stays in the upper vagina, where it dissolves slowly. Occasionally a woman will be allergic to the bioadhesive tablet. Vagifem raises the blood level of estradiol less than 5 percent after the vagina has thickened from its use.

Estring is a very low dose vaginal bioidentical estradiol ring that has almost only a local effect in the vagina. It is a good choice for women who cannot take systemic estrogen and do not want an atrophic vagina. It also lasts three months, just like the Femring.

Estrogen Dosing

The dosage for estrogen replacement should be based on symptoms and blood tests. The same plan can be used for women who have not had a hysterectomy but will be using cycled or continuous progesterone or progestin to prevent endometrial cancer. There are many clinical scenarios, and I will review a few of the most common.

Surgical Menopause

A pre-menopausal woman who has just had her uterus and ovaries removed will require the immediate replacement of estrogen to avoid severe hot flashes. Any woman who underwent a hysterectomy should have had sequential compression devices employed during surgery to prevent blood clots in her legs, but she is still at risk postoperatively and should not be given oral estrogen until about two weeks after the procedure. I prefer Vivelle Dot 0.1 mg twice-weekly patches or Climara 0.1 mg once-weekly bioidentical estradiol patches. These are usually applied the evening or morning after surgery. This dose is continued until the two-week postoperative visit, at which time other alternatives are discussed if needed. At six weeks, an estradiol level is obtained and the dosage is adjusted to be between 50 pg/ml and 150 pg/ml. If a 0.1 mg bioidentical estradiol transdermal patch does not prevent estrogen deficiency symptoms, then two patches may be used at once. An extra patch is added until symptoms are relieved. A hot flash is the brain screaming out for glucose because it is starving, as there is not adequate estrogen to facilitate glucose transport across the blood-brain barrier. Hot flashes are not funny. Some women have required as many as four 0.1 mg estradiol patches before menopausal symptoms were controlled. Their estradiol levels were about 60 pg/ml with four 0.1 mg patches. They chose to change to compounded bioidentical estradiol lotion, which can be made in any strength, to decrease their costs. Most young women usually require .075 mg or .1 mg patches for adequate replacement. Some young women do very well on .0375 mg bioidentical estradiol patches with relief of symptoms and excellent estradiol levels. The goal is to use the lowest dose that relieves symptoms of estrogen deficiency (vaginal dryness, hot flashes, night sweats, or other vasomotor symptoms) and gives a physiologic estrogen level (50 pg/ml to 150 pg/ml, or up to 40 pg/ml to 160 pg/ml if needed). Estradiol replacement should be continued throughout life.

A woman over one year into menopause and having hot flashes should be given estrogen in a rapidly increasing dose until her symptoms are relieved. If samples are available, I dispense one week of bioidentical estradiol .05 mg patches and see her weekly until symptoms are relieved. An estradiol level will be done when symptoms have resolved. If symptoms are not relieved with 0.1 mg patches, then two 0.1 mg patches are used. If this relieves her symptoms, then the dose is decreased weekly (0.1mg+0.1mg, then 0.1mg+. 075mg, then 0.1mg+. 05mg, then 0.1mg+. 0375 mg) until symptoms return. The dose is then increased to the dose at which symptoms did not occur and kept at that level. The required dose will usually decrease as the body gets used to the lower dose and liver metabolism of estrogen slows. Vagifem vaginal bioidentical estradiol tablets twice weekly are begun at the first visit if she has vaginal dryness symptoms. The Vagifem can usually be discontinued after the first or second kit of fifteen tablets has been taken, as the vagina will stay healthy from the transdermal bioidentical estradiol dose.

If a woman is less than two years into menopause and wants oral estrogen, she should start estradiol 0.5mg, Premarin or Cenestin 0.3mg and increase the dose weekly until symptoms are relieved. The required dose varies widely, and a few women will require a lower dose. If generic estradiol is used, changes in symptoms and blood levels must be followed closely. If the patient begins using a product made by a different generic company, blood levels should be retested. As most of the estradiol is converted into estrone as it passes through the liver, estradiol and estrone levels should be checked to know the ratio of estradiol to estrone. The sum of the estradiol and the estrone should be about 100 pg/ml to 300 pg/ml.

Women experiencing menopause but not having hot flashes should slowly start estrogen replacement. A normal-size woman would start using .0375 mg bioidentical estradiol patches, check her estradiol level in three weeks, adjust the dose up one level until the estradiol level is 50 pg/ml to 150 pg/ml, and ensure there are no symptoms of estrogen excess or deficiency. Divigel, Estrogel, Elestrin or Estrasob would also be good bioidentical estradiol choices. The starting dose would be one pump of Estrogel or Elestrin or one packet of Divigel or Estrasorb. The dose would be increased one pump or packet monthly until normal estradiol levels are reached and symptoms are relieved, and then that dose would be continued for life. Evamist is a spray bioidentical estrogen that you start with one spray daily and increase by one spray weekly or monthly depending on symptoms and estradiol levels.

Oral estrogens, such as estradiol, Femtrace, Estrace, Premarin, Cenestin or others, should be started at a low dose and increased monthly based on symptoms and findings regarding adequate estrogen replacement. Estradiol and estrone levels can be checked after clinical relief of estrogen deficiency is achieved. Some women will feel wonderful and have very high estrogen levels even with the lowest dose pill and will need some other route of replacement.

The Femring is another excellent bioidentical estradiol alternative, especially for women allergic to adhesives or sensitive to changes in estrogen levels. It only comes in two doses, .05 mg and .1 mg bioidentical estradiol per day, which may be too much or too little for some women, but most women will find one of these doses to be adequate. The ring is inserted vaginally and then changed every three months. Estrogen levels go up for one to two days and then level out and remain at basically the same level for the next three months. In most women—even women who have not ever been pregnant—it fits in the vagina well and is not noticeable to them or their partner.

Compounded bioidentical estradiol lotion is an excellent alternative for women who are allergic to adhesives or have reasons they cannot take oral hormones, such as the Femring not fitting or the smallest dose patch being too strong or the largest dose patch being too weak. Some women simply prefer to use compounded lotion–based bioidentical estradiol, and testosterone or progesterone can be added if necessary. Compounded bioidentical estradiol lotion will be covered in detail in another chapter.

Hormones for Women Who Have Not Had a Hysterectomy

Women who have not had a hysterectomy (removal of the uterus with or without the ovaries) need the same estrogen replacement as women who have had a hysterectomy. In addition, they also need continuous or cycled progesterone or progestin treatment to prevent endometrial cancer. The endometrium is the inside lining of the uterus. Before menopause occurs, there is a large surge of progesterone after ovulation during each cycle to ready the lining of the uterus for implantation and early development of a pregnancy. If a pregnancy does not occur at this time, then progesterone levels fall rapidly on days twenty-seven and twenty-eight of the cycle, and the thick lining is shed to get ready for the next month. The progesterone also helps the nuclei of the endometrial cells to mature, preventing endometrial cancer. When a woman does not ovulate, progesterone is not produced, and the endometrial cells age. A woman who does not ovulate regularly is at increased risk for endometrial precancer (called endometrial hyperplasia) and endometrial cancer. When pregnant, a woman produces huge quantities of progesterone, and as would be expected, the more pregnancies a woman experiences, the lower her risk of endometrial cancer. Birth control pills stop ovulation, but they also deliver a daily dose of progestin in sufficient amounts to prevent endometrial cancer. Women on the birth control pill who take cycled, extended-cycle, or continuous daily pills for over ten years have an 80 percent decrease in their risk of endometrial cancer.

During the 1970s, in order to decrease the risk of endometrial cancer seen with continuous estrogen use, women were cycled with ten to thirteen days of a progestin monthly, duplicating the natural monthly cycle of progesterone. This worked well, but few women liked having periods monthly after menopause, so other alternatives were studied. The current literature supports a program of two weeks of progesterone or progestin exposure three or four times a year to significantly reduce the risk of endometrial cancer. In nature, the purpose of the monthly progesterone cycling is to prepare the body and the uterus for pregnancy. Because we are only trying to prevent endometrial cancer, not prepare for pregnancy, three or four cycles a year is adequate. No one method seems to be perfect, but any unscheduled bleeding should be evaluated with a vaginal ultrasound and an endometrial biopsy with local anesthesia to detect precancer before cancer develops.

The package inserts of estrogen products says that estrogen can increase the risk of endometrial cancer. Indeed it can, if a progestin or progesterone is not taken along with it for years. The typical woman diagnosed with endometrial cancer is a woman in her 60s, 70s, or 80s who never took hormones and is suffering from postmenopausal bleeding. Taking hormones properly prevents most endometrial cancer!

A woman in menopause with or without hot flashes who has not had a hysterectomy may already have unrecognized endometrial problems. A vaginal ultrasound should be done either in the first few weeks after starting hormones or before starting hormones, to confirm there is a normal, thin endometrium (uterine lining) without any trapped mucous or blood in the uterus. A pelvic exam should be done at the same time frame to identify vaginal or cervical problems. If there is a problem and it is not identified, then women and their families may blame symptoms on the hormones. In fact, it is the hormones that help to identify the problem in this case. The choice of the type of estrogen used and the method of delivery in this case is the same as that of a woman who has had a hysterectomy. After a physiologic level of estrogen is achieved, then cycled progesterone or progestin treatment is begun.

Oral cycled progesterone or progestin options:

> Prometrium 200mg (micronized, natural, bioidentical progesterone)
>
> Aygestin 5mg (norethindrone acetate)
>
> Provera 10mg (medroxyprogesterone acetate)

All of these are taken for fourteen days every three or four months, fourteen days every two months, or twelve days every one month depending upon how often a woman wants to have a period. The period that follows is usually like the period that a woman had when she was younger, although it is frequently lighter because the total dose of hormones given is less than most women produce before menopause. Taking the progestin or progesterone for the first twelve or fourteen days of the month puts the period midmonth, not at the end of the month. Most holidays fall at the end of the month, so most women prefer this. It is usually easier for women to remember the first of the month, so they often use that to help them start the hormone on time. It is impractical to manufacture a transdermal patch for the delivery of progesterone. The patch would have to be very large. Progestin is a much more potent drug that acts on the endometrial lining in the same way as progesterone, and it can be administered transdermally.

Transdermal cycled progestins:

> Combipatch 50/250
>
> ClimaraPro .045/.015

Both of these patches give bioidentical estradiol and a progestin daily. More women tolerate this regimen to protect the endometrium than any other. If a postmenopausal woman is on twice-weekly bioidentical estradiol patches and her therapeutic dose is less than bioidentical estradiol.05 mg (50 mcg) per day, then the Combipatch 50/250 is *substituted* for the bioidentical estradiol patch twice weekly for two weeks every one, two, three or four months, depending on a woman's desired frequency of periods in order to protect her from endometrial cancer. If her bioidentical estradiol dose is 50 mcg per day or more, then the Combipatch 50/250 is *added* to the bioidentical estradiol patch for those two weeks.

ClimaraPro .045/.015 has a little less bioidentical estradiol, but about one-half as much progestin as Combipatch 50/250. To use ClimaraPro as cycled therapy, two patches must be used together per week for two weeks to get enough progestin to cause the endometrium to mature.

Progesterone in lotion can be used to cycle as well, but high concentrations must be used in order to get enough progesterone through the skin to mature the lining of the uterus. A compounding pharmacy can prepare progesterone 6,000 mg mixed in 30 ml of propylene glycol and added to nine ounces of Jergens lotion (remove one ounce of lotion from a ten-ounce bottle). The bottle must be shaken very well before each use. One teaspoon of the lotion is rubbed into the abdomen, thighs, or buttocks (never the breasts) every day for fourteen days every one to four months. Progesterone lotion is a bioidentical transdermal solution to progesterone supplementation.

Transvaginal progesterone is available as a commercial product and gives a very nice maturation effect on the endometrium. Crinone or Prochieve is the brand name, and they are sold as 4 percent and 8 percent gels. The 8 percent gel is for use daily from day eighteen of the cycle until ten to twelve weeks into gestation to support a pregnancy in women who do not make enough progesterone. Crinone or Prochieve 4 percent gel is sold in kits of six applicators to be used only every other night for twelve nights to induce maturation of the lining. When this is used only every four months, many women tolerate it well and prefer it.

Progesterone can also be given as a compounded vaginal suppository. Progesterone suppository 25mg nightly the first 14 days of January, May and September can be used. Some women prefer Progesterone 50 mg suppository every other night for 7 suppositories the first 14 days of January, May and September. Both methods give 14 days of progesterone to mature the lining and will be followed by a period.

Another transvaginal option is the Nuvaring. The Nuvaring is a vaginal contraceptive ring that doses a woman with one-half the dose of the lowest-dose birth control pill. It provides enough estrogen to be adequate for most women and enough progestin to protect women from endometrial cancer. It is sold to be used for three weeks, but it delivers a steady state of estrogen and progestin for more than one month. The Nuvaring can be used three months each year (January, May, September) for the entire month and then an estrogen replacement of a woman's choice can be used the rest of the year. This prescription regime, as well as most other progesterone supplement regimens, is not approved by the FDA but has been very useful for women who do not like or do not tolerate other methods of receiving progesterone or progestins.

Women who prefer the Femring for estrogen replacement find the Nuvaring very convenient. They use the Femring for three months and then the Nuvaring for one month, having three usually small periods each year. Theoretically the Nuvaring should provide adequate estrogen replacement. Some women require other estrogen, in addition to the Nuvaring, to prevent menopausal symptoms.

Continuous Combined Hormone Replacement Therapy for Women Who Have Not Had a Hysterectomy

Many women do not like having periods during menopause. In order to prevent endometrial cancer and not have periods, continuous combined hormone replacement therapy was studied from the late 1970s into the early 1980s. Enough evidence was available to start using it safely in the early 1980s, and it has been used since. Any estrogen regimen (pills, patches, gels, lotions, or vaginal rings) can be used with daily adequate progestin as a continuous combined regimen. There are also several commercial combined products; premixed and compounded combined lotion can be used as a continuous regimen as well.

Continuous progestin and progesterone regimens require the progestin and progesterone to be taken daily in addition to whatever estrogen is being used. This is not how the body gives progesterone. The surge in progesterone after ovulation is what causes premenstrual syndrome (PMS) in many women. Some women who take continuous progesterone will have continuous PMS.

If there are no contraindications, then the following oral progesterone or progestins can be used:

Prometrium (bioidentical progesterone) 100 mg daily

Aygestin (norethindrone acetate) 2.5 mg daily

Provera (medroxyprogesterone acetate) 2.5 mg or 5.0 mg daily.

There are also combined estrogen and progestin products made in pills and patches. The pills are taken daily, providing estrogen and progestin in one pill.

Activella (1 or 0.5mg bioidentical estradiol and 0.5 or 0.1mg norethindrone acetate) comes in two combinations. The original strength 1/0.5 mg pills may be cut with a pill cutter to get the right dose and save money. If 1mg estradiol is not enough, then either two Activella can be taken or an additional bioidentical estradiol pill of 0.5 mg or 1 mg can be taken with the Activella.

PremPro is a combination of conjugated equine estrogen and medroxyprogesterone acetate that comes in several different combinations (.3 mg/1.5 mg, .4 mg/1.5 mg, .625 mg/2.5 mg, and .625 mg/5.0 mg). Dosing of PremPro, Premarin, and Cenestin is done clinically based on how a woman feels and what her exam shows. The lowest dose PremPro is begun and then it is increased every one to two weeks until symptoms, if any, are relieved. If there are no hot flashes, then the dose is increased monthly until physical examination shows adequate estrogen effect.

Continuous Combined Patches

Two patches are available for continuous combined therapy. Combipatch 50/140 is applied twice weekly or ClimaraPro .045/.015 is used weekly. If the estradiol level is not adequate, increasing to the Combipatch 50/250 will raise the estradiol level. If the estradiol level is still not adequate, then an estrogen patch can be added to the combined patch.

For women who should not take pills and cannot use patches or would prefer daily lotion, a continuous combined regimen that works for most women can be compounded of estradiol and progesterone. This is compounded in Jergen's lotion or any other high-quality lotion of a woman's choice. The prescription is:

Estradiol _____mg

And

Progesterone _____mg mixed well in one ounce of propylene glycol.

Remove one ounce of lotion from a ten-ounce (8 to 16oz) bottle of Jergen's lotion (or any lotion of the patient's choosing). Add, and mix in well, the estradiol/progesterone/propylene glycol to make a full bottle.

The prepared lotion should be dispensed from the original lotion bottle, which should be labeled appropriately.

Directions: Rub in ½ tsp (2.5 ml) daily to the skin of the lower abdomen, buttocks, and thighs.

Using ½ tsp daily should allow this bottle to last about four months. It is not critical to use exactly 2.5ml. About the same amount should be used every day. Some women prefer to use 1 tsp; this will cause the bottle to last two months. The usual starting dose when ½ tsp is used is estradiol 100 mg and progesterone 1,000 mg. The target amount of estradiol in the blood test is still 50 pg/ml to 150 pg/ml, and the goal for the progesterone level is 2 ng/ml (1.8 to 2.4). The initial dose is started, and dosing size is adjusted as needed based on symptoms. After four to six weeks on the same dose, estradiol and progesterone blood levels are obtained, and dosages are adjusted in the next bottle. An average woman undergoing menopause has thirty-five or more years to adjust the dose, so there is no rush except when symptoms are present. It is better to adjust the dose stepwise over several bottles rather than jump to the predicted dose unless there are hot flashes. Increasing hormone doses too fast can cause too many side effects. The average dose needed is 300 mg estradiol and 3000 mg progesterone, but the doses required have varied as much as one hundred times to achieve physiologic hormone levels.

The goal in successfully implementing continuous combined hormone replacement therapy is for no bleeding to occur. Breakthrough bleeding occurs in more than one-half of women using continuous combined HRT. If it is not too bothersome, it will usually stop during the first six months of replacement. If it has not stopped by that point, then a cause for the bleeding should be investigated. Many women on continuous combined HRT will have breakthrough spotting or bleeding after not bleeding for months before. If no endometrial biopsy has been done in the last two years, a vaginal ultrasound and endometrial biopsy under local anesthesia should be done to check for pre-malignant or malignant changes of the endometrium. When breakthrough bleeding occurs changing the ratio of estrogen to progestin by giving extra estrogen for one week can frequently control it. This can be with an extra bioidentical estradiol patch 0.1mg for one week or with oral bioidentical estradiol 2mg, Premarin 1.25mg or estrone 1.25mg twice daily for 1 week. This brief rise in estrogen stimulates growth of the stromal cells that support the blood vessels and glands of the endometrium. If bleeding persists after two treatments in one week, then further evaluation—usually a hysteroscopy—will diagnose and treat the cause of the bleeding in most women. Continuous combined replacement works well for many women. If irregular bleeding or progesterone-related symptoms make this treatment intolerable, cycled hormone replacement or the Mirena intrauterine system should be considered. Many, if not most, women will have less bleeding when cycled three times yearly then if they try to have no periods with continuous combined hormone replacement therapy.

Mirena is a progestin-releasing IUD, or intrauterine device. It is the only progestin source that has not had patients develop endometrial hyperplasia (precancer) or endometrial cancer occur while using it. It is inserted and left in place for ten years in menopause. It is only manufactured in one factory in Finland. The FDA only approves it for five years. There has to date not been a case of endometrial hyperplasia (precancer) or endometrial cancer in a patient with the Mirena in place. The Mirena placement, like the endometrial biopsy, should be done with local anesthesia. The local anesthesia dramatically increases patient acceptance and patient referrals for Mirena. Endometrial cancer is the most common gynecologic cancer in women in the United States. If all women in menopause had a Mirena placed under local anesthesia and changed every ten years then this would almost or completely eliminate endometrial cancer. Women are only waiting for the FDA to approve this so it will be a covered benefit. (Do not hold your breath!)

Testosterone Replacement for Sex Drive

Estradiol is made from testosterone in the ovaries. Testosterone is produced by the ovaries and the adrenal gland. Pre-menopausal women's testosterone levels range from 20 ng/dl to 50 ng/dl for most of the month. On days eleven and twelve of a normal menstrual cycle, there is a two-day surge in testosterone levels that happens every month. This surge in testosterone levels is extremely necessary in some women for an adequate libido (sex drive). Of course, other factors are also important; if that were not the case, every young woman would have an inappropriate sex drive when she started her periods. Testosterone injections have been used for decades to increase sex drive in women and men with low libido. Testosterone levels are high for most of the month in these people, but the libido is only high for one to two weeks after the injection. In addition, this prolonged elevation of testosterone can cause excess hair growth and acne in many women. Trying to talk women out of using testosterone injections while the injections are working is usually unsuccessful. The women said they would take care of the extra hair growth and acne; they just wanted their injections. In order to mimic the natural two-day surge in testosterone, 4 percent testosterone cream was tried. The cream had been used for skin conditions in the past. The cream was inconsistent, and many women did not like the feel of the cream. Topical compounded testosterone in propylene glycol given for two days once monthly gives an excellent surge in testosterone and at some dose will almost always markedly increase libido. Some women also need a two-day surge in estrogen with the testosterone in order to experience the same effect. This mimics the natural two-day surge of estrogen and testosterone that every woman has every month before ovulation unless she is on birth control pills or not ovulating for other reasons. If a woman loses her sex drive because of birth control pills, then this two-day surge of testosterone will frequently return it. Testosterone supplementation, even for two days, can rarely increase hair growth on the face and other places in women. This problem occurs much less often with two-day-per-cycle supplements than with daily testosterone supplements or monthly testosterone injections.

Dry Eyes

In addition to sex drive, testosterone will also frequently help return moisture to dry eyes in postmenopausal women. Recent studies have shown that the Meibomian glands at the base of each eyelash that lubricate the eyes only have testosterone receptors.[37] Studies have also shown that postmenopausal women on estrogen alone have an increased risk of dry eye syndrome. Women or men with dry eye syndrome will have to use lubricating eye drops every fifteen to sixty minutes while awake and every one to two hours while asleep. Some women with excellent baseline testosterone levels may still develop dry eye syndrome. Most women with adequate estrogen replacement levels will convert enough back into testosterone to have excellent baseline levels. Two groups of women—those women who were given two days of testosterone a month, and those women who had testosterone injections to increase libido—reported that their dry eyes had incidentally improved. After examining this situation, it was found that women with dry eye syndrome who were given two-day transdermal testosterone supplements during menopause experience 60 to 100 percent relief. Although these are clinical observations based on basic science and anatomy, they must be confirmed by more scientific study. However, by duplicating normal physiology, the monthly two-day surge in testosterone both increased sex drive and improved dry eyes in most women.[38]

Summary

1. The WHI ignored the natural history of breast cancer and heart disease.

2. Breast cancer is diagnosed earlier in women who take estrogen and progestin. Women who do not take estrogen are just as likely to develop breast cancer as those who do within one to two years.

3. In the WHI studies, there was no new breast cancer.

4. The risk of dying from breast cancer is decreased in women taking hormones according to most studies published.

5. The WHI ignored the pharmacology of conjugated equine estrogen and medroxyprogesterone acetate and the relative reasons not to take them orally.

6. The risk of heart disease is decreased if hormones are begun at menopause and continued for life.

7. Women with risk factors for heart disease should use transdermal or transvaginal estrogen (and progestin if needed).

8. Cardiac benefits of restarting estrogen should not be expected for fifteen years based on the natural history of heart attacks.

9. Hormones reduce the risk of hip and other fractures. Hip fracture is much more painful and debilitating, and has a worse prognosis, than breast cancer.

10. The risk of Alzheimer's disease is significantly reduced with estrogen use.

11. The risk of nursing home placement (loss of independence) is significantly reduced with estrogen use.

12. Hot flashes are a symptom of the brain starving and should be stopped with estrogen replacement if possible.

13. Estrogen decreases the risk of death from all causes by 33 to 37%.

14. The risk of dying from a heart attack is reduced by 53% with estrogen use.

15. The risk of dying from all cancers is reduced by 29% with estrogen use.

16. Women with a mother or sister with breast cancer will experience a 35% reduction in dying from all causes with estrogen use.

17. Women in all risk groups will experience a significant reduction in the risk of dying with estrogen use.

18. Estrogen treatment should be started at menopause and continued for life.

19. Estrogen treatment can be started at any age to prevent estrogen deficiency and can be continued for life.

20. Estrogen dosage is based on levels, symptoms, and physical findings.

21. Women with a uterus in place who are taking estrogen should take continuous or cycled progesterone or progestins to prevent endometrial cancer.

22. Transdermal testosterone replacement should be given for two days monthly to help sex drive and possibly prevent or treat dry eye syndrome.

23. Taking women off estrogen therapy to reduce their risk of health problems is just as absurd as castrating men to improve their health.

    (Women should never be taken off estrogen except for those with breast cancer or metastatic endometrial cancer.)

24. Stopping estrogen therapy upon admission to the hospital or for surgery is not justified. Switching to transdermal or transvaginal estrogen from oral estrogen should be considered in any woman at risk for clots.

Conclusion

The WHI ignored the natural history of breast cancer and heart disease. Breast cancer must grow for almost seven years before it is large enough to be seen on mammography. It is three more years before the breast cancer is large enough (1 cm) to be palpated. Coronary heart disease develops when a fifteen-year-old cholesterol plaque ages and its surface cracks. In the WHI study, there were no new cases of breast cancer. There were a few cases of breast cancer that grew faster in women on hormones, but the rate of diagnosis of breast cancer was the same in both groups. Not taking hormones did not prevent or decrease the risk of breast cancer.

Prescribing oral hormones to women at risk for a heart attack or stroke ignores the pharmacology of oral conjugated equine estrogen and medroxyprogesterone acetate. Hormones begun at menopause and continued for life decrease the risk of heart attack but should not be used to treat or prevent heart disease. Heart disease should be prevented by lifestyle modifications and appropriate preventive supplements. If a woman has risk factors for heart disease or cerebrovascular disease, she should use transdermal or transvaginal estrogen and progesterone (or progestin). Postmenopausal hormones dramatically decrease the risk of hip and other fractures. Hip fractures are much more painful and debilitating than breast cancer, and they have a worse prognosis. Twenty-five percent or more of women who suffer a hip fracture will never walk independently again. Fifteen to twenty percent will die in the first year.

The risk of developing Alzheimer's disease is reduced (four to six times) with estrogen use. Alzheimer's disease is prevented, but not treated, with estrogen replacement. Hot flashes, flushes, hot feelings at night, and night sweats are symptoms of the brain starving in response to estrogen deficiency. Nursing home placement, with loss of independence, is significantly increased in women not taking estrogen. This increase is due to a higher occurrence of Alzheimer's disease, osteoporosis, hip fractures, spinal fractures, and heart attacks.

Estrogen decreases the risk of dying from all causes 33 percent to 37 percent. The risk of dying from a heart attack is reduced 53 percent with estrogen use. The risk of dying from all cancers is reduced 29 percent in women on estrogen. Women with a mother or sister with breast cancer experience a 35 percent reduction in all causes of death when they take estrogen. Women in all risk groups experience a significant reduction in the risk of dying with estrogen use.

Women who have had a hysterectomy should start estrogen at menopause and continue estrogen use for life. The dose is determined by symptoms, physical findings, and blood tests. Women who have not had a hysterectomy should start using estrogen and progesterone (or progestin) at menopause. Cancer of the endometrium (the inside lining of the uterus) is the most common cancer of the female organs. The risk of getting endometrial cancer is decreased by using cycled or continuous progestin or progesterone with estrogen. Estrogen and progesterone (or progestin) should be continued for life.

Sex drive (libido) can be restored in many women with two days of transdermal testosterone mimicking the two-day surge of testosterone women have on days eleven and twelve of every menstrual cycle. A two-day surge of testosterone also reverses dry eye syndrome in many women. Studies will, with hope, show it prevents dry eye syndrome as well.

Women should stop estrogen use at whatever age it is recommended that men be castrated to improve their health. Women should not stop using estrogen if they develop an illness unless men are castrated for that illness. Women with breast cancer should stop using estrogen until they have reviewed for themselves the literature on taking estrogen after the diagnosis of breast cancer.

No estrogen or estrogen-level test is being sold by the authors of this book. What is being sold to women are their lives, that they may take them back from the statisticians, epidemiologists, and news media that have mislead them, their families, their friends, and their physicians. What can women do to correct this? Women who have suffered and people who have seen their loved ones suffer should write letters and fax them to their senators to demand that the H.E.L.P. Committee of the U.S. Senate hold hearings to review the WHI and WHIMS conclusions. Also, they should write and fax their U.S. representatives to demand that the U.S. House of Representatives Committee on Energy and Commerce hold similar hearings. The H.E.L.P. Committee of the U.S. Senate and the Committee on Energy and Commerce of the U.S. House of Representatives are responsible for the National Institutes of Health and the WHI. Women will continue to suffer, become disabled, and die prematurely because of the NIH until the incorrect conclusions of the WHI and WHIMS studies are corrected.

Have strength, demand the estrogen you or your loved ones need and deserve, and fight to correct this ignorant and arrogant attack on the health and lives of women.

Financial disclosure and conflicts: Blane Crandall has received speaker fees and training from Pfizer and Novartis. He has never received a grant or salary from the NIH.

www.menopausefree.org

Donna Walters

My website is a quick overview of some of the positive results from taking estrogen and lists some interesting information relative to estrogen use. I am concerned with the wild disorder associated with the estrogen environment which began as a result of the WHI study. I have waited for eight years for someone to challenge the results of that study and the harm and fear it's created. Sadly, the wait continues. I feel that until someone stands up — albeit someone prepared to be battered and tossed around in that out-of-control environment — nothing will change. So, I am tossing my hat in the ring for the sole purpose of gathering strength in numbers and standing up for the millions of women who are tired of not having important medical information that is needed, both accurate and timely, to enable them to make the right decisions concerning their health. With that statement — let the time be now and count me in for the long haul ahead!

In an attempt to prevent another WHI boondoggle from ever occurring again, my website has three hyperlinks for the purpose of recording important information, which I am hopeful women will provide.

1. One hyperlink will record the information of women who have taken estrogen for longer than twenty years. To my knowledge, this will be the first database recording the observational information of long-term estrogen users.

2. The second hyperlink will record the information of women who have suffered any type of medical consequences as a result of the inaccuracy of the WHI study. Again, to my knowledge, there is no such database presently receiving any type of observational information of medical consequences suffered as a result of the erroneous WHI study results as announced.

3. The third hyperlink asks women if they would like to be part of the estrogen awareness effort and sign a petition that will be used for the purpose of getting legislation introduced in order to make it mandatory that all future federally funded estrogen studies must have the study data independently verified before the results can be disclosed to the public. This will ensure that the pandemonium resulting from the WHI study will never occur again. The WHI study was supposed to provide important medical information concerning estrogen and help women make decisions concerning estrogen use. The study was costly ($735 million) and none of the objectives were attained; one cannot help but wonder whether the funds were spent in the best possible way to benefit women's health.

Hopefully, over time I will hear from many women regarding this subject, as I believe our health issues should be given a higher priority than what we have seen in the past. The estrogen pandemonium is dangerous today because women are left with more questions than answers, and yet there is nothing on the horizon that is going to change or provide those much-needed answers in order for women to obtain the best of health.

There is strength in numbers, and with that in mind, I hope women will lend me their support in an attempt to start the work necessary to modify and resolve these much-needed health issues for the good of all women:

♀ Estrogen has been in the marketplace for sixty-three years and not *one* improvement or modification has taken place, which is amazing considering all the advances made by science in that time.

♀ The number one cause of death among women is heart disease, and yet *nothing* has changed in this area either.

♀ Women are responsible for many things in the course of their lifetimes: the marriage; family; and in today's society, a career. When those responsibilities are over and women reach their golden years, what does a woman have to look forward to? Heart disease; osteoporosis; menopause; the loss of her femininity, sex appeal, and pleasant attitude; her body being stretched from childbearing; weight gain from menopause; hair loss; and wrinkles. No, I don't believe that is a good reward or a satisfactory state to be in at the average age of fifty when, according to today's life expectancy figures, women have another twenty or more years of life and productivity ahead of them. At this same age, men are still very much in the game of life. The window of opportunity is now open for women to remain in the game along with their counterparts.

Women must begin to change some of the undesirable past medical situations, and I, for one, am ready to work in that direction and am hopeful that my example can be a starting point.

Please join me in getting the word out to all women who are stuck in the fear of the 2002 WHI inaccurate announcement. Let's educate those who have not yet done the vital research in order to make an informed decision according to the most recent studies on hormone replacement therapy. We will be doing a world of good for our sisterhood.

Bibliography

Writing Group for the Women's Health Initiative Investigators, "Risks and benefits of estrogen plus progestin in healthy postmenopausal women. Principal results from the Women's Health Initiative randomized controlled trial," JAMA 288 (2002): 321–333.

Collaborative Group on Hormonal Factors in Breast Cancer, "Breast Cancer and hormone therapy: collaborative reanalysis of data from 51 epidemiologic studies of 52,705 women with breast cancer and 108,411 women without breast cancer," Lancet 350 (1997): 1047–1059.

Grady, D., D. Herrington, V. Bittner, et al., for the HERS Research Group, "Cardiovascular disease outcomes during 6.8 years of hormone therapy: Heart and Estrogen/Progestin Replacement Study Follow-up (HERS II)," JAMA 288 (2002): 49–57.

Espeland, M, S. Rapp, S. Shumaker, et al., for the Women's Health Initiative Memory Study Investigators, "Conjugated equine estrogens and global cognitive function in postmenopausal women. Women's Health Initiative Memory Study," JAMA 201:2959–2968.

Endnotes

[1] Robert A. Wilson, MD, FICS, FACS, FACOG, *Feminine Forever*, New York: Evans (with Lipincott), 1966.

[2] Writing Group for the Women's Health Initiative Investigators, "Risks and benefits of estrogen plus progestin in healthy postmenopausal women. Principal results from the Women's Health Initiative randomized controlled trial," JAMA 288 (2002): 321–333.

[3] The Women's Health Initiative Steering Committee, "Effects of conjugated equine estrogen in postmenopausal women with hysterectomy," The Women's Health Initiative Randomized Controlled Trial. JAMA 291 (2004): 1701–1712.

[4] Burkman, R. T., J. A. Collins, and R. A. Greene, "Current perspectives on benefits and risks of hormone replacement therapy," Am J Obstet Gynecol 185(2) (2001): S13–S23.

[5] Tang, M. X., Jacobs, Stern Y, et al., "Effect of oestrogen during menopause on risk and age at onset of Alzheimer's disease," Lancet 348 (1996): 429–432.

[6] Zandi, P. P., M. C. Carlson, B. L. Plassman, K. A. Welsh-Bohmer, L. S. Mayer, D. C. Steffens, and J. C. S. Breitner, "Hormone replacement therapy and incidence of Alzheimer disease in older women The Cache county study," JAMA 288 (2002): 212–329.

[7] Nanda, K., L. A. Bastian, and K. Schulz. "Hormone replacement therapy and the risk of death from breast cancer: a systematic review." Am J Obstet Gynecol 186(2) (2002): 325–34.

[8] Ries, L. A. G., D. Harkins, M. Krapcho, A. Mariotto, B. A. Miller, E. J. Feuer, L. Clegg, M. P. Eisner, M. J. Horner, N. Howlader, M.

Hayat, B. F. Hankey, and B. K. Edwards, eds, "SEER Cancer Statistics Review, 1975-2003," National Cancer Institute, http://seer.cancer.gov/csr/1975_2003/, based on November 2005 SEER data submission, posted to the SEER website 2006.

[9] American Heart Association, *Heart Disease and Stroke Statistics-2005 Update*, Dallas, Texas:American Heart Association.

[10] Speroff, L. and M. A. Fritz, *Clinical gynecologic endocrinology and infertility-7th ed.*, 2005; 16:610.

[11] Wertheimer, M. D., M. E. Costanza, T. F. Dodson, C. D'Orsi, H. Pastides, and J. G. Zapka, "Increasing the effort toward breast cancer detection," JAMA 255 (1986): 1311–1315.

[12] Vuster, V., L. Badimon, J. J. Badimon, and J. H. Chesebro, "The pathogenesis of coronary artery disease and the acute coronary syndromes," N Engl J Med. 326 (1992): 242–250.

[13] Speroff, L. and M. A. Fritz, *Clinical gynecologic endocrinology and infertility-7th ed.*, 2005; 18:689–777.

[14] Collaborative Group on Hormonal Factors in Breast Cancer, "Breast cancer and hormone therapy: collaborative reanalysis of data from 51 epidemiologic studies of 52,705 women with breast cancer and 108,411 women without breast cancer," Lancet 350 (1997): 1047–1059.

[15] Psaty, B.M., S. R. Heckbert, D. Atkins, R. Lemaitre, T. D. Koepsell, P. W. Wahl, D. S. Siscovick, and E. H. Wagner, "The risk of myocardial infaction associated with the combined use of estrogens and progestins in postmenopausal women," Arch Intern Med. 154 (1994): 1333–1339.

[16] Heckbert, S. R., N. S. Weiss, T. D. Koepsell, R. N. Lemaitre, N. L. Smith, D. S. Siscovick, D. Lin, and B. M. Psaty, "Duration of estrogen replacement therapy in relation to the risk of incident myocardial infarction in postmenopausal women," Arch Intern Med. 157 (1997): 1330–1336.

[17] Grodstein, F., J. E. Manson, and Stampfer, "Postmenopausal hormone use and secondary prevention of coronary events in the nurses' health study. A prospective observational study," Ann Intern Med. 135 (2001): 1–8.

[18] Wood, D., G. D. Backer, O. Faergeman, et al., "Prevention of coronary heart disease in clinical practice: Recommendations of the Second joint task force of European and other societies on coronary prevention," Eur Heart J. 19 (1998): 1434–1503.

[19] Huley, S., D. Grady, T. Bush, et.al., for the Heart and Estrogen/progestin Replacement Study (HERS) Research Group, "Randomized trial of estrogen plus progestin for secondary prevention of coronary heart disease in postmenopausal women," JAMA 280 (1998): 605–613.

[20] Grady, D., D. Herrington, V. Bittner, et al., for the HERS Research Group, "Cardiovascular disease outcomes during 6.8 years of hormone therapy: Heart and Estrogen/Progestin Replacement Study Follow-up (HERS II)," JAMA 288 (2002): 49–57.

[21] Sarrel, P. M., "The differential effects of oestrogens and progestins on vascular tone," Hum Reprod Update 5 (1999): 205–209.

[22] Baumgartner, M.R., J. H. Chrostowski, and R. N. Levy, "Intertrochanteric hip fractures," Chapter 48 in *Skeletal trauma: fractures, dislocations, ligamentous injuries 2nd ed*, (Philadelphia, Saunders).

[23] Surveillance, Epidemiology, and End Results (SEER) Program (www.seer.cancer.gov) SEER*Stat Database: Incidence - SEER 9 Regs Public-Use, Nov 2004 Sub (1973–2003), National Cancer Institute, DCCPS, Surveillance Research Program, Cancer Statistics Branch, released April 2006, based on the November 2005 submission.

[24] Mulnard, R. A., C. W. Cotman, C. Kawas, C. H. Van Dyck, et al, "Estrogen replacement therapy for treatment of mild to moderate Alzheimer's disease: a randomized controlled trial. Alzheimer's disease cooperative study," JAMA 283 (2000): 1007–1015.

[25] Wang, P. N., S. Q. Liao, R. S. Liu, C. Y. Liu, et al, "Effects of estrogen on cognition, mood, and cerebral blood flow in AD: A controlled study," Neurology 54 (2000): 2061–2066.

[26] Henderson, V. W., A. Paganini-Hill, B. L. Miller, R. J. Elble, et al., "Estrogen for Alzheimer's disease in women: Randomized,

double-blind, placebo-controlled trial." Neurology 54 (2000): 295–301.

[27] Ropper A. H. and R. H. Brown, *Adam's and Victor's principles of neurology, 8th ed.* 2005; 898–906.

[28] Wolfson, C., D. B. Wolfson, M. Asgharian, C. E. M'Lan, T. Østbye, K. Rockwood, and D. B. Hogan, for the Clinical Progression of Dementia Group, "A reevaluation of the duration of survival after the onset of dementia," N Engl J Med 344:1111–1116.

[29] Bishop, J, and J. W. Simpkins, "Estradiol enhances brain glucose uptake in ovariectomized rats." Brain Research Bulletin 36 (1995): 315–320.

[30] Observation of author.

[31] Rapp, S., M. Espeland, S. Shumaker, et. al., for the WHIMS Investigators, "Effect of estrogen plus progestin on global cognitive function in postmenopausal women. The Women's Health Initiative Memory Study: A randomized controlled trial," JAMA 289 (2003): 2663–2672.

[32] Shumaker, S, C. Legault, L. Kuller, et.al., for the Women's Health Initiative Memory Study Investigators, "Conjugated equine estrogens and incidence of probable dementia and mild cognitive impairment in postmenopausal women. Women's Health Initiative Memory Study," JAMA 291 (2004): 2947–2958.

[33] Espeland, M., S. Rapp, S, Shumaker, et.al., for the Women's Health Initiative Memory Study Investigators. "Conjugated equine estrogens and global cognitive function in postmenopausal women. Women's Health Initiative Memory Study," JAMA 291 (2004): 2959–2968.

[34] Ettinger, B., G. D. Friedman, T. Bush, and C. P. Quisenberry Jr., "Reduced mortality associated with long-term postmenopausal estrogen therapy." Obstet Gyenecol 87 (1996): 6–12.

[35] Grodstein, F., M. J. Stampfer, G. A. Grodstein, et al., "Postmenopausal hormone therapy and mortality." N Engl J Med 336 (1997): 1769–75.

[36] Speroff, L., and M. A. Fritz, *Clinical gynecologic endocrinology and infertility-7th ed.,* 2005; 6:195.

[37] Sullivan, D.A., B. D.Sullivan, J. E. Evans, F. Schirra, H. Yamagami, M. Liu, S. M. Richards, T. Suzuki, D. A. Schaumberg, R. M. Sullivan, and M. R. Dana, "Androgen deficiency, Meibomian gland dysfunction, and evaporative dry eye syndrome," Ann NY Acad Sci. 966 (2002): 211–222.

[38] Personal observation.

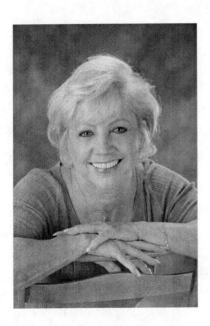

Donna Walters

Donna Walters was born in Texas. Her father was an Air Force officer and pilot in World War II and after returning from a tour in Germany, the family settled in the suburbs of Washington D.C. where Donna spent the majority of her life. Donna attended Trinity University in Washington, D.C., majoring in Business Administration. She has been married for more than forty-three years and has three children and five grandchildren.

Donna worked on Capitol Hill for almost ten years in a variety of Congressional staff positions, including secretary to several individual Members of Congress. Her last position was a Subcommittee Clerk for the Subcommittee on Oceanography, House Committee on Merchant Marine and Fisheries, which included taking roll call votes of the Members during legislative markup sessions. Following her Congressional service, Donna worked as support staff in the White House for approximately four years. In the Carter administration, Donna worked with the Office of Correspondence and in the West Wing with the Deputy Assistant for Domestic Policy and, on occasion, with

President Carter's Chief of Staff. During the Reagan administration, Donna worked with the Office of Presidential Personnel and the Office of Correspondence.

After leaving the White House, Donna worked with partners in various law firms for the past twenty years and has experience in the areas of intellectual property, trusts and estates, lobbying, and corporate law. She was the assistant to the managing partner in the District of Columbia office of an international law firm, assistant to the managing partner of a large Virginia based law firm, was the Senior Corporate Assistant in the corporate and securities practice in the Virginia office of a global top fifteen law firm. Presently Donna is an assistant with the second largest law firm in the United States.

Donna has been actively involved in her husband's business for more than fifteen years handling all of the administrative tasks required of a small business with annual gross revenues in excess of one million dollars.

Donna was also active in her community's youth organization serving on their Board of Directors for more than ten years, developing and expanding various sports program for young girls. She also served as a team representative on the Northern Virginia Swimming League for approximately seven years.

Donna enjoys writing, sports and traveling.

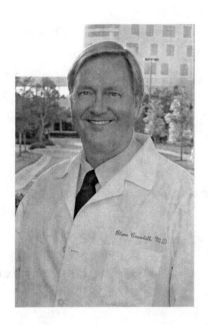

Dr. Blane Milton Crandall

A physician truly dedicated to the well being of each individual patient, Dr. Blane Milton Crandall is uniquely qualified to evaluate hormone issues for women. He was raised in a medical family. His father was a primary care physician in Melbourne, Florida, and Blane accompanied him as early as age 4 to house calls, nursing home and hospital visits. By age 14 Blane decided that he would become a physician. He was accepted in the early admissions program to Emory University. He was also accepted in the early admissions program to medical school at Emory University School of Medicine. While at the School of Medicine he was awarded the Evangeline Papageorge Award for outstanding service to the university.

A recurring theme in his life has been service; service to his community, service to his university and after medical school at the end of the Viet Nam War, Dr. Crandall served his country during his Family Practice Residency at Silas B Hays Army Medical Center at Ft. Ord, California. In 1979 he returned to his hometown in Melbourne to join his father's practice. He was among the first group of physicians

Board Certified in the specialty of Family Practice. Not satisfied with the limitations of the specialty of Family Practice, he applied for a second residency in Obstetrics and Gynecology in 1984.

By 1984 Dr. Crandall had been married for sixteen years and had four children. He completed his Obstetrics and Gynecology Residency training at the acclaimed Madigan Army Medical Center in 1987 and served his country as Chairman of the Department of Obstetrics and Gynecology with the 101st Airborne Division in Ft. Campbell, Kentucky. Since his move to Naples, Florida, in 1989, Dr. Crandall has been the recipient of numerous civic and professional awards and served as Chairman of the Department of Obstetrics and Gynecology at Naples Community Hospital for two terms. He has been selected by his peers as one of the "Best Doctors in America" every year since 1999.

He has traveled to Washington D.C. four times since the release of the Women's Health Initiative in 2002 to speak with our legislators regarding issues on women's health.

In his thirty year career as a physician, Dr. Crandall has treated more than 50,000 postmenopausal women. He has written numerous articles on Hormone Replacement Therapy and has been a national speaker on the subject. His experience, education and passion for excellence in healthcare uniquely qualify him to comment on the medical issues of women in America.

LaVergne, TN USA
23 September 2010
198072LV00003B/5/P